100 Questions About Allergies

Jonathan Corren, MD
Allergy Medical Clinic, Research Division
Los Angeles, California

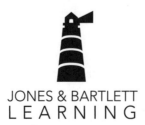

JONES & BARTLETT
LEARNING

World Headquarters

Jones & Bartlett Learning
40 Tall Pine Drive
Sudbury, MA 01776
978-443-5000
info@jblearning.com
www.jblearning.com

Jones & Bartlett Learning
Canada
6339 Ormindale Way
Mississauga, Ontario L5V 1J2
Canada

Jones & Bartlett Learning
International
Barb House, Barb Mews
London W6 7PA
United Kingdom

Jones & Bartlett Learning books and products are available through most bookstores and online booksellers. To contact Jones & Bartlett Learning directly, call 800-832-0034, fax 978-443-8000, or visit our website, www.jblearning.com.

Substantial discounts on bulk quantities of Jones & Bartlett Learning publications are available to corporations, professional associations, and other qualified organizations. For details and specific discount information, contact the special sales department at Jones & Bartlett Learning via the above contact information or send an email to specialsales@jblearning.com.

The author, editor, and publisher have made every effort to provide accurate information. However, they are not responsible for errors, omissions, or for any outcomes related to the use of the contents of this book and take no responsibility for the use of the products and procedures described. Treatments and side effects described in this book may not be applicable to all people; likewise, some people may require a dose or experience a side effect that is not described herein. Drugs and medical devices are discussed that may have limited availability controlled by the Food and Drug Administration (FDA) for use only in a research study or clinical trial. Research, clinical practice, and government regulations often change the accepted standard in this field. When consideration is being given to use of any drug in the clinical setting, the healthcare provider or reader is responsible for determining FDA status of the drug, reading the package insert, and reviewing prescribing information for the most up-to-date recommendations on dose, precautions, and contraindications, and determining the appropriate usage for the product. This is especially important in the case of drugs that are new or seldom used.

Production Credits
Executive Publisher: Christopher Davis
Editorial Assistant: Sara Cameron
Production Director: Amy Rose
Associate Production Editor: Jessica deMartin
Associate Marketing Manager: Marion Kerr
Manufacturing and Inventory Control
  Supervisor: Amy Bacus
Composition: Glyph International
Printing and Binding: Malloy, Inc.

Cover Credits
Cover Design: Carolyn Downer
Cover Printing: Malloy, Inc.
Cover Images: Woman in hat: © olly/Shutter-
Stock, Inc.; Bowl of nuts: © Elena Elisseeva/
Dreamstime.com; Bee and flower: © manfredxy/
ShutterStock, Inc.; Girl with dog: © Photodisc;
SEM of pollen: Courtesy of Louisa Howard
and Charles Daghlian, Dartmouth College,
Electron Microscope Facility

Library of Congress Cataloging-in-Publication Data
Corren, Jonathan.
  100 questions & answers about allergies / Jonathan Corren.
    p. ; cm.
  Other title: 100 questions and answers about allergies
  Other title: One hundred questions & answers about allergies
  Other title: One hundred questions and answers about allergies
  Includes index.
  ISBN 978-0-7637-7609-1 (alk. paper)
  1. Allergy—Miscellanea. 2. Allergy—Popular works. I. Title. II. Title:
100 questions and answers about allergies. III. Title: One hundred questions
& answers about allergies. IV. Title: One hundred questions and answers
about allergies.
  [DNLM: 1. Hypersensitivity—Examination Questions. WD 300 C824z 2011]
  RC585.C67 2011
  616.97—dc22

2010011061

6048

Printed in the United States of America
14 13 12 11 10   10 9 8 7 6 5 4 3 2 1

To my father and mother, who provided me with the quiet inspiration to pursue a career in medicine.

Contents

Walking through the park on a sunny spring day, playing with your pet dog, or eating peanuts at a baseball game represent some of life's greatest pleasures. However, each of these activities can turn into uncomfortable, or even life-threatening, events if you happen to be allergic. The allergic diseases have a tremendous impact on society, as they are among the most common of all medical conditions and continue to increase each year. During the past 20 years of clinical practice, including work at an academic medical center as well as a private practice, I have diagnosed and treated a large number of patients with these diseases. As my patients learned to live with these chronic disorders, they challenged me with questions, ranging from why they had their particular problem to what the best cure might be. In this book, I present the answers to these questions, based on my experience and lessons learned from the world's scientific literature.

Part One addresses general issues regarding allergic diseases, focusing on definitions of these diseases, what is responsible for recent increases in prevalence, and who is most susceptible to developing them.

Part Two turns to the topic of nasal allergy. This section is the largest in the book, as it covers an extremely common condition and one that many patients attempt to treat on their own. The first set of questions revolve around the diagnosis of nasal allergy, including a review of the substances that cause allergy as well as which diagnostic tests are most accurate. This is followed by an analysis of existing therapies, ranging from over-the-counter medications to alternative treatments to therapies offered only by allergy specialists. This section goes on to discuss disorders that often coexist with nasal allergies, such as sinusitis and nasal polyps, as well as how to handle nasal allergy in special situations, including pregnancy and airplane flights.

The book then offers important information on the most frightening of allergic disorders, those that result in serious and even life-threatening systemic reactions. These include allergy to foods (Part Three), insect stings (Part Four), and drugs (Part Five). In these sections, the most important aspects of anaphylaxis are explored.

In the sixth and final section of the book, allergic skin diseases are reviewed, including atopic dermatitis, contact dermatitis, and hives.

Readers of this book may notice that there is no discussion of asthma, which is a very important and increasingly common allergic disorder. Asthma is covered in two other books in the 100 Questions & Answers series, one about asthma in general and the other regarding asthma in children.

It is my hope that the information presented in this book will assist patients in knowing when to seek medical advice about their allergies, and which diagnostic tests and treatments are most beneficial.

Jonathan Corren, MD

General Concepts in Allergy

What are the allergic diseases, and how common are they?

What has caused the recent increase in allergic diseases?

When do allergies usually come on, and will they go away during adulthood?

More . . .

1. What is an allergy?

Allergy

A type of hypersensitivity reaction to environmental substances caused by IgE antibodies.

Antibody

A protein formed by the immune system that helps protect the body from infection and is also responsible for certain types of hypersensitivity reactions.

Immunoglobulin E (IgE)

The antibody that is responsible for allergic responses.

Mast cell

A type of tissue cell rich in histamine, which is the major cause of immediate allergic reactions.

Histamine

A compound released during allergic reactions that causes capillary dilation, smooth muscle contraction, and sensory nerve stimulation.

Leukotriene

A family of lipid molecules, which are released during allergic reactions and whose most prominent effects are tissue swelling and bronchoconstriction.

The word **allergy** refers to a reaction to an environmental substance, either by breathing it, eating it, or having contact with the skin. The most common mechanism by which an environmental substance causes this kind of reaction involves **antibodies**, which are proteins formed by the immune system. The normal function of antibodies is to protect the body from infection by attacking and killing organisms like viruses and bacteria. In the case of allergy, the antibody is called **immunoglobulin E**, or IgE, and, rather than attaching itself to microorganisms, the antibody binds to normally harmless substances like pollen, dust mites, and animal danders. Once IgE is formed in the bloodstream, it seeks out and binds to a type of cell called a **mast cell**, which is located in the mucous membrane of the eyes, nose, lungs, and gastrointestinal tract as well as skin. If the person is then reexposed to that same allergen, the mast cell is triggered within a few minutes to release a variety of chemicals, including **histamines**, **leukotrienes**, and **prostaglandins** (**Table 1**). These chemicals, which are also referred to as mediators of the allergic response, are responsible for the symptoms that patients develop after exposure to allergens.

Table 1   Chemicals Involved in Allergic Reactions

Chemical	Target Organ	Effects
Histamine	Nose, eyes, lungs	Nasal itch, sneezing, nasal discharge, itch and redness, wheezing
Leukotriene D_4	Nose, lungs	Nasal congestion, discharge, wheezing
Prostaglandin D_2	Nose	Nasal congestion, eye itch, wheezing

2. What are the allergic diseases, and how common are they?

The primary allergic diseases include allergic asthma, allergic rhinitis, atopic dermatitis, anaphylaxis, and food hypersensitivities (**Table 2**).

Asthma is a disease of the lungs in which the bronchial mucous membrane is chronically irritated and inflamed. This inflammation makes the airways more hyperreactive to a variety of provocative stimuli, including allergens, cold air, exercise, and viral infections, leading to bronchospasm. Typical symptoms include wheezing, chest tightness, cough, and shortness of breath, which may occur episodically or continuously. The disease is diagnosed by history, findings on examination, and pulmonary function testing.

Allergic rhinitis (to be discussed in greater depth later) is similar to asthma, in that it represents mucosal inflammation of the nose. The most common symptoms are nasal congestion, sneezing, itching, and discharge. The diagnosis of rhinitis is based primarily upon the history and physical examination.

Prostaglandin

A family of lipid molecules derived from arachidonic acid whose effects include tissue inflammation.

Asthma

Disease of the lungs in which the bronchial mucous membrane is chronically irritated and inflamed. The hallmarks of this disease include episodic, reversible spasm of the airways in response to both specific (e.g., allergens) and nonspecific (e.g., cold air) triggers.

Allergic rhinitis

Mucosal inflammation of the nose due to an allergic reaction.

Table 2   Primary Allergic Diseases

Disease	Symptoms
Allergic rhinitis	Sneezing, itching, discharge, congestion
Anaphylaxis	Hives, flushing, sneezing, nasal discharge, throat swelling, wheezing, nausea, vomiting, diarrhea, dizziness, fainting
Asthma	Wheezing, chest tightness, shortness of breath, cough
Atopic dermatitis	Patches of itchy red skin, most often in creases of the extremities
Food allergy	Any of the above

Atopic dermatitis

A chronic eczematous skin disease characterized by redness, itching, and scaling.

Atopic dermatitis is an eczematous skin disease that usually begins in infancy and is characterized by redness, itching, and scaling (see Question 95). It most commonly affects the flexural areas of the arms and legs.

Anaphylaxis

A life-threatening allergic reaction most often involving the skin (hives), lungs (wheezing), and circulation (low blood pressure).

Anaphylaxis is a life-threatening condition in which a systemically administered allergen, such as a food, drug, or insect sting triggers the rapid and massive release of mast cell mediators throughout the body. The ensuing reaction may involve the skin, airways (including nose, larynx, and lungs), gastrointestinal tract, and systemic circulation, with symptoms of flushing, hives, wheezing, throat swelling, dizziness, or even loss of consciousness.

Food hypersensitivity

An adverse immunologic response to a food protein.

Food hypersensitivity includes a variety of hypersensitivity reactions, most commonly including IgE-mediated anaphylaxis and aggravations of atopic dermatitis (see Question 52).

3. Has there been an increase in allergic diseases?

Over the past 2 decades, a significant portion of the world, particularly the United States, western and northern Europe, Canada, Australia, and New Zealand, has witnessed a substantial increase in allergic diseases. Approximately 2 decades ago, 3% of the American population had asthma; today the prevalence is closer to 7%. Similarly, during the same time span, the prevalence of allergic rhinitis has increased from 10% to 20%; for atopic dermatitis, prevalence has increased from 5% to 8%; and for anaphylaxis, prevalence has increased from 1% to 3%. This point is brought home even more dramatically by a large national study, called the National Health and Nutrition Examination Survey (NHANES); in 2008, 58% of Americans tested positive for at least one airborne allergen.

4. What has caused the recent increase in allergic diseases?

These alarming increases are not completely understood. However, one popular explanation has been labeled the hygiene hypothesis. This theory stipulates that all humans are born with an allergic predilection. As growing infants encounter new environmental challenges, such as viruses and bacteria, their immune systems shift away from the allergic profile toward one that is capable of protecting them from infectious organisms.

Agricultural environments, with the presence of animal fecal material, have proven to be particularly instrumental in helping young immune systems mature away from their allergic origins. In less developed countries around the world, there is still extensive exposure to fecal-derived microorganisms at an early age, resulting in a relatively low prevalence of allergic problems. In the United States, Canada, New Zealand, and the countries of western and northern Europe, children have been increasingly raised in urban, nonagricultural settings in which they are raised apart from other children. This lack of exposure to agricultural animals and manure as well as a lower prevalence of viral upper respiratory infections have been associated with an increased prevalence of allergic diseases.

Another important contributor to the rising prevalence of allergies may be nutrition. Countries with high rates of diseases such as asthma and allergic rhinitis have lower blood levels of certain vitamins, including vitamins C and D. Vitamin D may be particularly important, as it is a critical component of a well-functioning immune system. Finally, pollution of indoor air (particularly cigarette smoke) and outdoor air have been shown to contribute significantly to the development of allergies and asthma.

5. If my spouse or I have allergies, what are the chances that our child will have allergies?

There is a strong genetic component in determining which individuals will develop allergy. If one parent has an allergic disease, including asthma, rhinitis, atopic dermatitis, or food allergy, there is an approximate 40% chance that the child will have some form of allergy; with both parents having an allergic disease, the risk rises to 60%. There are a large number of genes that contribute to this risk of allergy.

6. When do allergies usually come on, and will they go away during adulthood?

Usually, eczema (atopic dermatitis) develops in the creases of the arms and behind the knees in the first year of life and signifies that a child will be an allergic individual. Approximately half of children with atopic dermatitis will go on to develop allergic rhinitis and/or asthma in the next 5 to 10 years. Of note, the vast majority of patients who develop an allergic disease will do so by age 30 years. Atopic dermatitis is the first problem to appear and also usually the first to resolve; by age 10 years, allergic eczema has resolved or improved markedly in up to 90% of children. Allergic rhinitis and asthma, once established, have a very low rate of remission.

PART TWO

Nasal Allergy

What factors in the environment trigger
nasal allergies?

What are allergy shots, and how effective
are they for nasal allergies?

Do nasal allergies worsen during pregnancy,
and how should they be treated?

More . . .

7. What are the symptoms of nasal allergies?

Patients with seasonal nasal allergies, also known as seasonal allergic rhinitis or seasonal hay fever, often have intermittent nasal symptoms that may become acutely worse while the patient is outside of the house, particularly if it is windy. Symptoms usually consist of some combination of sneezing, itching of the nose, nasal discharge, and congestion. Sneezing may occur in bouts of 5 to 10 or more sneezes that occur sporadically throughout the day. Itching will frequently lead the patient, especially children, to push the nose upward in a repetitive pattern ("allergic salute"). The discharge may come out of the nostrils or may drip down the throat; it is most often clear in color and thin and watery in consistency. If the mucus becomes very thick and starts to acquire a yellowish or greenish color, one must suspect the possibility of an infection. Congestion is a prominent symptom in half of all patients with nasal allergies and is due to a combination of swollen membranes and mucus trapped in the nose. In addition to these four major nasal symptoms, about half of patients with seasonal allergy also have eye symptoms, which consist of itching, redness, and watering.

As symptoms persist during a several week-long allergy season, constant rubbing around the eyes may lead to redness and a thickened appearance of the skin. Along with all of these symptoms, a number of other complaints such as headaches, facial pain, ear blockage, and cough, may also be very bothersome. This constellation of seasonal allergy symptoms differs somewhat from patients that have year-round allergic rhinitis, particularly when the allergy is caused by house dust mites. In mite-allergic patients, congestion is usually the biggest complaint, and eye symptoms are much less common.

8. How can I tell if I have allergies or colds?

Symptoms of allergies and colds can be quite similar, but there are some differences that will help distinguish them (see **Table 3**). With regard to the types of symptoms, both allergies and colds cause symptoms of sneezing, congestion, and runny nose. However, colds are more likely to begin with fever and sore throat before the gradual onset of these other symptoms, while in allergic rhinitis, these symptoms come on quickly without any fever or throat pain. Specific symptoms may vary as well; colds often cause a yellowish discharge by the seventh day of the infection, while allergies are much more likely to cause thin, watery nasal secretions. In addition, itching of the eyes and nose may be very prominent with allergies but virtually absent with a common cold. With respect to the duration of symptoms, colds generally last from 5 to 7 days, whereas allergy symptoms continue as long as a person is exposed to the allergy-causing agent. In addition, allergy symptoms may subside soon after elimination of allergen exposure.

Allergies and colds cause symptoms of sneezing, congestion, and runny nose. However, colds are more likely to begin with fever and sore throat.

Table 3   Is It a Cold or an Allergy?

Parameter	Cold	Allergy
Fever	Often	No
Sore throat	Often	Unusual
Sneezing	Often	Often
Runny nose	Often	Often
Color of discharge	Clear, yellow	Clear
Itching of nose	No	Often
Itching of eyes	No	Often
Duration	7–10 days	Persistent
Season of year	Often in winter	Spring, summer, and fall; or year-round

Finally, the time of year may provide a helpful clue. Colds are much more likely to occur in the colder winter months, while allergies occur sporadically throughout the entire year or may be most prominent during the spring, summer, and/or fall seasons.

9. What factors in the environment trigger nasal allergies?

The most important allergens that cause allergic rhinitis are airborne substances. These airborne allergens can be divided into those that are present only seasonally versus those that are present year-round (also called "perennial"). Seasonal allergens are generally present in the outdoor environment and include tree, grass, and weed pollens as well as outdoor molds. In the United States, tree pollen can usually be found in the early spring (February through April), grass pollen in the summer months (May, June, and July), and weed pollen in the late summer and early fall (August, September, and October). All of these plants produce small and light pollen granules that can be carried through the air for miles as compared with fruit- and flower-bearing plants, which rely upon insects for pollination. Outdoor molds, the most common of which are *Cladosporium* and *Alternaria*, can often be found in the outdoors in high levels throughout the year, but peak levels usually occur in the late summer and fall, particularly in the Midwest. Perennial allergens are usually found indoors and include house dust mites, animal fur or skin, indoor molds (like *Aspergillus* and *Penicillium*), and cockroaches. Food allergy is not a common cause of nasal allergies and is more likely an issue in young children who also have eczema. However, certain foods and beverages, particularly alcohol, may cause **vasodilation** of the blood vessels in the nose, which leads to nasal congestion.

Vasodilation
The widening of blood vessels.

10. I work in an office building with sealed windows, and my nasal symptoms seem worse while I'm there. Could the building be responsible?

Many patients note that their symptoms mainly occur, or worsen, while they are at work. This condition is referred to as **occupational rhinitis**. The most common causes of work-related symptoms are airborne irritants. Common examples of irritants in the workplace include wood dust (carpenters), paper dust (office workers), textile dusts (clothing manufacturers), smoke (firefighters), cleaning fluids (janitors), quick-drying glues (furniture makers), and paint (painters). It is important to know that these substances do not cause true allergic reactions, and therefore suitable skin and blood allergy tests cannot be performed. Common examples of true allergens that cause rhinitis in the workplace include animal fur (laboratory workers and veterinarians), wheat flour (bakers), and plant pollens (gardeners).

Occupational rhinitis

Rhinitis that is associated with an individual's work environment.

11. When I'm exposed to perfume, my nose runs. Is this an allergy?

There is a large group of people, probably constituting 50% of patients with chronic nasal symptoms, who develop a watery nasal discharge and/or stuffiness when they are around certain nonallergenic nasal triggers. This nasal disorder is called **nonallergic rhinitis**, and the triggers that are most commonly reported include cold air, airborne irritants (e.g., perfume, paint fumes), weather changes, and spicy foods. In the case of spicy foods, it is important to note that the food is not acting as an allergen and will not provoke more severe symptoms such as throat swelling or wheezing upon future exposure.

Nonallergic rhinitis

Nasal inflammatory disease that is not caused by IgE-mediated hypersensitivity to allergens.

Perfume, like many other scented products, is a volatile organic compound (VOC), which, at room temperature, evaporates very quickly and enters the air as small particles. It is important to know that this irritant effect is not due to an allergy to perfume, and there is no skin test or blood test that can demonstrate that a person has a sensitivity to these things. When patients with this problem can anticipate that they will be exposed to a known trigger, such as perfume, they can take ipratropium bromide nasal spray 0.03% (two sprays per nostril 15 to 20 minutes beforehand) to block the development of symptoms. In patients with chronic, daily symptoms of nonallergic rhinitis due to frequent exposure to known triggers, azelastine hydrochloride nasal spray, used on a regular basis, may also be very effective.

12. Does drinking milk increase nasal mucus production?

It has been a widely held belief that drinking milk or eating dairy-containing foods causes an increase in nasal mucus production. However, there is no scientific evidence that daily consumption of milk has a chronic effect on nasal mucus production. Milk can act as an allergen in children (usually younger than 5 years) and occasionally older children and adults. Milk allergy usually manifests with gastrointestinal symptoms, including diarrhea or cramping; as a skin rash, with eczema or hives; and less commonly with anaphylaxis, consisting of throat swelling, wheezing, and/or low blood pressure. If you suspect that a member of your family does not tolerate milk in some way, bring it to the attention of your physician and inquire whether an allergic evaluation would be beneficial. Because milk is a very important source of vitamins A and D, riboflavin, calcium, and protein, I recommend against removing milk and other dairy products from their diet without medical consultation.

13. I've been using Afrin nasal spray daily for the past 6 months to treat my stuffy nose. Why do my symptoms seem to be getting worse?

Frequently, patients with nasal congestion caused by an acute upper respiratory infection or nasal allergies will treat themselves with an over-the-counter nasal decongestant spray such as Neo-Synephrine (phenylephrine) or Afrin (oxymetazoline). While short-term use of these medications, on the order of 3 to 5 days, is generally considered safe, when patients use the sprays for longer periods of time, they frequently develop rebound nasal congestion. This problem is referred to as **rhinitis medicamentosa**, which, if not treated properly, may worsen. As the rebound congestion becomes more severe, many people simply increase the amount of the decongestant nasal spray to treat their escalating symptoms. Occasionally, patients end up using their decongestant spray on an hourly basis, waking up at night multiple times in order to use the medication. At this point, patients will require regular treatment with an intranasal corticosteroid spray for several weeks and will need to have the underlying cause of their original nasal symptoms addressed. If topical nasal corticosteroids are not effective, oral steroids may be needed for several days while the nasal tissue heals.

Rhinitis medicamentosa

Rebound nasal congestion brought on by extended use of topical nasal decongestants.

14. Do alcohol, tobacco, marijuana, and cocaine have any serious effects on the nose?

Alcoholic beverages, regardless of type, dilate blood vessels throughout the body, including the nose, and frequently cause an increase in nasal congestion. In addition, alcohol is dehydrating and may lead to a thickening of nasal secretions. It does not generally lead to other symptoms, such as sneezing, itching, or nasal discharge.

The effect of alcohol is transient and is usually recognized by the patient after multiple experiences. In rare cases, a patient may be allergic to a component in the beverage, such as hops or yeast, which may trigger nasal symptoms as well as other systemic complaints.

Smoking tobacco, whether it be in the form of cigarettes, cigars, or water pipes, has also been observed to contribute to nasal symptoms. It is speculated that the tars and products of combustion act as irritants to the mucous membrane, leading to increases in congestion, sneezing, and nasal secretions. While it is unlikely that patients are allergic to the tobacco itself, the dried leaves may contain appreciable amounts of various types of mold, which may act as respiratory allergens in sensitized individuals. Similar comments may be made regarding marijuana, which can act as a potent irritant and trigger of nasal symptoms but is unlikely to act as an allergen.

Cocaine is most frequently used intranasally, and many chronic users complain of nasal irritation, nasal crusting, recurrent nosebleeds, nasal stuffiness, and facial pain. The most likely source of these symptoms is the constriction in blood vessels in the mucous membrane and septum, which may ultimately result in a perforation or hole in the septum (so-called "coke nose"). Because nasal congestion is a common complaint in cocaine users, many self-treat with nasal decongestants, such as oxymetazoline, which adds to the problem because it also leads to the constriction of blood vessels.

15. I was told that I have a deviated septum and that this makes my allergies worse. Do I need to have it surgically repaired?

Nasal septum

The small cartilaginous structure that divides the nose into halves.

The **nasal septum** is the small cartilaginous structure that divides the nose into halves (**Figure 1**). Approximately

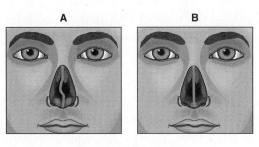

Figure 1   Nasal septum: (A) deviated; (B) normal.

one-third of people have deviation of the septum toward one side of the nose or the other. This condition is either present from birth or is caused by trauma later in life. The external nose may look completely normal without any obvious deformity, or the nose may look shifted to one side. The vast majority of individuals who have a nasal septal deviation have no symptoms attributable to the deviation, and it is only detected during a routine physical examination. A minority of patients, however, will notice blockage of the nose, with one side being significantly and consistently more blocked than the other side. Additionally, when the patient lies down, the sensation of obstruction becomes much worse due to the effects of gravity upon blood flow through the nose. An isolated nasal septal deviation will not cause other nasal symptoms such as nasal discharge, itching of the nose, or sneezing.

A useful test in the office is to spray both sides of the nose with oxymetazoline topical decongestant nasal spray and wait 10 minutes. If the patient's nasal congestion improves markedly on both sides of their nose, it would indicate that nasal swelling, rather than septal deviation, is the most prominent problem and should be dealt with prior to considering surgical intervention. If the deviation is extremely severe, with the septum touching the turbinates and resulting in complete blockage on that side of the nose, the patient can be referred to a head and neck surgeon for surgical repair of the septum (referred to as septoplasty).

In the case of patients with mild to moderate deviations of the septum and concomitant allergic rhinitis, a good approach is to first treat the rhinitis as completely as possible, including both allergen avoidance measures and anti-allergy medications. If, after a 1-month trial of treatment, the patient has minimal symptoms of congestion, the septal deviation will not require surgical correction. However, if the patient continues to notice bothersome one-sided nasal blockage on the side of the deviation, he or she is a good candidate for septoplasty. Patients should always ask exactly what procedures the surgeon is planning to perform. If the major anatomic problem is the septal deviation, then other nasal structures, such as the **turbinates** and **paranasal sinuses** (see Question 44), should be left undisturbed. Once the nose has undergone surgery, it is very difficult to reverse those changes.

Turbinate

A long, narrow, and curled bone that comes off of the lateral wall of the nasal passage and is important in the humidification, filtration, and warming of inspired air.

Paranasal sinuses

The air-filled spaces within the bones of the skull and face.

16. What causes chronic nasal blockage in infants?

Infants younger than 1 year of age frequently have signs of nasal blockage, most often because of thick secretions that are stuck in their nose. Other symptoms, such as sneezing or ocular symptoms, are much less common in very young children. This problem has been referred to as "rhinitis of infancy," which is almost universally related to exaggerated physiologic mucus production that cannot be effectively cleared from the nose. Often, the symptoms are most prominent after a viral upper respiratory tract infection and may last for several days to a few weeks following the infection. As the internal dimensions of the nose grow larger, these symptoms usually improve, and by 1 year of age, they may have completely resolved.

This problem is best treated with saltwater flushes and a bulb aspirator to remove the secretions. If the nasal discharge is yellow or green, the baby may have developed bacterial sinusitis following a cold, which may require oral antibiotics for satisfactory recovery. Hypersensitivity to airborne allergens is rare at 6 months of age and does not usually begin until 1 to 2 years of age. Infants may have a food allergy at this age, but this most often presents with eczema, which is a red, itchy, scaly rash; gastrointestinal symptoms; and is a rare cause of isolated nasal symptoms in infants.

17. I started to have a stuffy nose in my late 60s. What is the most likely cause?

Chronic nasal complaints developing later in life are usually not allergic in origin. The most likely causes of new-onset rhinitis in patients older than 60 years of age includes nonallergic rhinitis, anatomic obstruction (such as a deviated septum or **concha bullosa**), drug-induced rhinitis (topical decongestants and some blood pressure medications), and rhinitis associated with systemic diseases (most commonly hypothyroidism).

In older patients, nonallergic rhinitis is frequently aggravated by dryness of the nasal membranes and loss of cartilage in the supporting structures of the nose. The loss of cartilage is due to a reduction in collagen protein synthesis, which is present throughout the body. This resultant sagging of the external portion of the nose further adds to the reduction in airflow through the nose. Treatment of nonallergic rhinitis in the elderly should generally include some form of nasal moisturization treatment, such as an over-the-counter nasal

Concha bullosa

An air pocket that occurs in the nasal turbinate bones, causing enlargement of the turbinate and often resulting in obstruction to airflow.

saline spray, and a medication. The two medications that have proven most effective for nonallergic rhinitis and that are approved by the U.S. Food and Drug Administration (FDA) for this indication are fluticasone propionate nasal spray, which is an intranasal steroid, and azelastine nasal spray. Both of these medications have been shown to reduce nasal congestion and discharge significantly. For patients who primarily have watery discharge without stuffiness, ipratropium bromide nasal spray is an effective alternative and has also been approved by the FDA for treatment of this symptom. Other medications, such as oral antihistamines, oral decongestants, and montelukast, have not been properly evaluated in patients with nonallergic rhinitis, and in my experience, have not been particularly helpful to these patients.

18. What is an allergy skin test?

To determine what a patient is allergic to, a physician will need to perform an allergy test. Allergy tests assess whether a patient has IgE antibodies (see Question 1) to a specific allergenic substance. The most commonly performed allergy test is the allergy **prick/puncture skin test**, in which a small amount of allergen solution is placed on the skin and a tiny sterile needle or plastic device is pricked or punctured through the skin. After waiting 15 to 20 minutes, the test is read by the physician or the physician's assistant. A positive test is signified by a small bump, also referred to as a wheal, surrounded by an area of redness, also called the "flare response," which is usually quite itchy. When physicians are attempting to determine whether a patient with suspected allergic rhinitis has an allergy and what substances should be avoided, a screening test, usually consisting of 10 to 15 allergens, is

Prick/puncture skin test

Allergy test in which the most superficial layer of skin is pricked or punctured with an allergen extract.

performed. Alternatively, if an allergy test is being conducted to create a therapeutic vaccine (allergy shots), anywhere from 50 to 70 tests are usually done, depending upon the geographic location where the patient lives. The prick/puncture skin test is highly reliable and accurate, and is considered the gold standard of allergy testing.

If the prick/puncture skin test is negative and allergies are highly suspected, the physician may elect to do additional testing using the **intradermal** method. This type of test is administered by injecting a small amount of allergen solution into the patient's skin and again waiting 15 to 20 minutes. A positive test requires the presence of both a wheal and a flare. While a negative intradermal test is very helpful in excluding an allergy to a given substance, a positive intradermal test is not particularly helpful, as many patients who are not actually allergic to a certain allergen may still show positive test results to that substance. For this reason, the intradermal test should only be performed and interpreted by physicians who are highly experienced in diagnosing allergic disease. Neither the prick nor the intradermal skin test can be performed in patients with diffuse skin disease or those who have taken a medication known to block the allergic response (most commonly antihistamines, such as Benadryl, or tricyclic antidepressants, such as doxepin).

The prick/ puncture skin test is highly reliable and accurate, and is considered the gold standard of allergy testing.

Intradermal test

An allergy test in which an allergen extract is injected into the skin.

Karen's comment:

I avoided going to the allergist for many years because I was afraid of having the skin test. I had scratch testing as a child, and it hurt for many hours afterward. My friend convinced me to do it and told me that it wouldn't be bad. It turned out that the way testing is done now just involves a light pricking of the skin compared with the old method where the skin was actually scraped and scratched. I didn't have any significant discomfort during the test, and it was not as painful as some blood draws that I've had.

19. What is an allergy blood test?

An alternative to allergy skin testing is blood testing, in which a small sample of a patient's blood is tested for the presence of IgE antibodies. In the past, the testing assay was based upon a radiolabeled technology called the **radioimmunosorbent test (RAST)**. More recently, laboratories have devised a new technique referred to as the ImmunoCAP test, which does not rely upon radioisotopes. The new test is considered quite accurate, but, compared with prick/puncture skin testing, it may miss up to 20% of IgE antibodies to selected allergens. Allergy blood tests can be performed even in the presence of skin disease, and the test results are not affected by drugs such as antihistamines. The most significant criticism of this type of testing is the higher cost and necessity of waiting several days to weeks for the results.

Radioimmunosorbent test (RAST)

A type of blood allergy test in which IgE antibodies to specific allergens are measured.

20. What are some alternative methods for diagnosing allergies?

Some laboratories offer a blood test that measures immunoglobulin G (IgG) antibodies to allergenic substances. IgG has never been demonstrated to be an important cause of allergic reactions; in fact, IgG may play a protective role in modulating the severity of allergic responses. IgG antibody tests have not been shown to accurately predict the occurrence of allergic reactions and have not proven useful in differentiating allergic from nonallergic individuals. For this reason, IgG antibody testing should not be used as a diagnostic laboratory test; nor should the results of these tests be relied upon to make recommendations for treatment.

End-point titration intradermal skin testing is an alternative method of skin testing that involves the injection of incrementally increasing concentrations of allergenic extracts. When these tests are positive at very low concentrations of allergen, the results are comparable to testing done by the prick/puncture method. However, when the tests are only positive at much higher concentrations of allergen, the results more likely represent false positives and do not accurately reflect true allergic sensitivity. For this reason, the prick/puncture method is the preferred testing modality.

21. What are the main steps in treating nasal allergies?

There are three basic steps to treating allergic rhinitis. The first step is to identify the allergens that the patient is sensitive to (by skin or blood testing) and institute measures for avoiding these allergens. There are specific, proven methods to reduce the levels of indoor allergens such as house dust mites, animal danders, indoor molds, and cockroaches. Exposure to outdoor allergens, such as plant pollens and outdoor molds, can only be reduced by staying indoors during peak hours (usually between 11 AM and 3 PM). If allergen avoidance does not adequately control nasal allergy symptoms, the next step is to add medications. There are several types of medications used to treat allergic rhinitis (**Table 4**), and in patients with moderate to severe symptoms, a combination of these drugs is often required. If allergen avoidance and medications are not successful in treating the rhinitis, allergen immunotherapy (allergy shots) is then typically recommended.

Table 4 Commonly Used Oral Antihistamines

Drug (Generic/Brand Name)	Generation/OTC	Child Dose	Adult Dose
Chlorpheniramine/ Chlortrimeton	Older/Yes	2 mg 2 × /d	4 mg 2 × /d
Diphenhydramine/ Benadryl	Older/Yes	12.5 mg 3 × /d	25 mg 3 × /d
Desloratadine/ Clarinex	Newer/No	2.5 mg/d	5 mg/d
Loratadine/Claritin	Newer/Yes	5 mg/d	10 mg/d
Cetirizine/Zyrtec	Newer/Yes	2.5 mg 2 × /d	10 mg/d
Levocetirizine/Xyzal	Newer/No	2.5 mg/d	5 mg/d
Fexofenadine/Allegra	Newer/No	30 mg 2 × /d	60 mg 2 × /d or 180 mg/d

22. If I keep a very clean house, do I need to worry about dust mites?

House dust mites, whose technical names are *Dermatophagoides pteronyssinus* and *Dermatophagoides farinae*, are microscopic insects that are relatives of the spider family. These tiny creatures are found throughout the world and live on a diet of sloughed human skin cells. An important component of their survival is a requirement of at least 45% relative indoor humidity. The primary reservoirs for dust mites are pillows, mattresses, bedding, upholstered furniture, and carpeting. The primary allergens of dust mites are proteins found in the body and fecal pellets of these insects. These allergenic mite proteins are bound to dust particles that are relatively large and heavy, preventing them from staying airborne for prolonged periods of time. Therefore, most of the exposure that occurs to dust mites occurs while an individual is lying in bed or on upholstered furniture. While it is very helpful to minimize surface dust in a person's home by vacuuming furniture and carpeting, this will not eliminate dust mites in a person's bed or in furniture cushions. This is best accomplished by placing plasticized cloth encasings over the pillow, mattress, and box spring and washing all linens in hot water (>130°F). Encasings that are labeled "hypoallergenic" but do not contain a plastic membrane will not effectively reduce exposure to allergenic mite proteins. If a person likes to lie down or sleep on couches and chairs, leather or vinyl upholstery is far preferable to cloth. **High-efficiency particulate air (HEPA) filters** have not been shown to reduce indoor dust mite levels or symptoms of mite-induced rhinitis.

23. If I have an allergy to mold, what can I do to prevent symptoms?

Fungi, which include thousands of different types of molds and yeasts, are a key part of the outdoor ecosystem. Molds are the fungal organisms to which most patients develop allergies. While many patients believe they have a mold allergy, the only way to confirm this sensitivity is through an allergy skin test (prick/puncture) or blood test for mold-specific IgE. These microscopic organisms typically consist of branching, filamentous structures, called "hyphae," along with small spherical structures, called "spores." Spores are released by molds into the air and are capable of traveling long distances. In a normal situation, most of the mold spores found inside a building come from the outdoor environment through doors and windows. Occasionally, the primary source of mold inside a dwelling may be water–damaged building materials caused by some type of leak.

People allergic to molds can take the following measures:

1. Stay indoors during periods when the outdoor mold spore counts are high. These outdoor counts can change quickly, and certain mold spores will increase in number during heavy winds (*Alternaria*, *Cladosporium*), while others will rise during damp periods

High-efficiency particulate air (HEPA) filter

A filter specially designed to remove greater than 90% of small (<1 micron) airborne particles.

Stay indoors during periods when the outdoor mold spore counts are high.

(*Aspergillus*, *Penicillium*). Most patients obtain information regarding mold counts by checking published reports; these data may need interpretation by an allergist to be useful.

2. Keep windows closed when outdoor mold spore counts are high. If this is not possible, an indoor HEPA filter may be helpful to remove spores from the indoor air. HEPA filters may be attached to the central heating and air conditioning system, or free-standing filtration units may be purchased. Electrostatic filters and devices that treat air with heat, ions, or ozone are not recommended.

3. Keep moist areas of the building, such as bathrooms and kitchens, well ventilated by keeping windows open and/or using an exhaust fan.

4. Maintain good building hygiene by cleaning carpeting, garbage pails, and refrigerators frequently and minimizing indoor plants with wet soil.

5. Keep indoor humidity below 45%. This may be challenging in areas with high humidity levels, such as areas by the ocean, lakes, or rivers, and may require the use of a dehumidifier. These devices should be drained and cleaned regularly. In addition, small space heaters or a low-wattage light bulbs may be useful in damp rooms or closets. Care should be taken to avoid creating a fire hazard.

6. Maintain building integrity by checking periodically for water leaks from defective roofing, windows, or plumbing.

7. Make corrections to drainage problems around and under the building. The landscape around the house should be properly graded to avoid movement of water from the surrounding ground toward the foundation, and dense plantings, leaves, and dead vegetation should be cleared from areas next to the building.

Taken together, these steps should be helpful in preventing outdoor and indoor mold exposure in mold-allergic patients.

24. If my child has nasal allergies, should we get rid of our cat?

While this question focuses on the role of cats in a patient's allergy, the information presented here is applicable to most furry pets, including dogs, rabbits, rats, and other small hairy or furry pets. An accurate history is the first step in determining whether a pet is the cause of someone's symptoms and whether removal of the pet will help. The most obvious question is whether symptoms worsen when the patient is close to or plays with the pet. If the answer to this question is yes, it makes the diagnosis of pet allergy. Occasionally, however, this question may not be helpful as some people own pets but do not have close contact with them. In that situation, it is important to ask whether symptoms increase when the patient is in the house, as well as whether symptoms improve when the person is away from the house for several days or longer.

Allergy testing to all relevant allergens is equally important in determining what the patient is allergic to, particularly when the initial questions do not yield clear-cut answers. In this case, either skin prick/puncture testing or blood allergy testing could be performed. However, if the blood tests are performed and are negative to all allergens, particularly the pet dander, I would recommend that skin testing be performed. If the skin testing is negative to the cat, there is no reason to remove the cat from the home. If the allergy test to the cat is positive, however, then the family is faced with a difficult choice. If the patient and family do not want to remove the pet from their home, and the patient's symptoms are minimal and stable, requiring either occasional or no medications, then I would cautiously recommend that the animal be allowed to remain in the house. In this case, a number of avoidance measures should be put into place, including preventing the pet from entering the patient's room; placement of allergen-barrier encasings on the pillow, mattress, and box spring; frequent vacuuming and damp-mopping of floors and hard surfaces; consideration of removal of the carpeting; and use of HEPA filters throughout the house. One research study revealed that compliance with these measures did reduce airborne pet allergen levels significantly.

If the patient's symptoms are more significant, and particularly if there is any degree of asthma present, I would strongly urge the family to give the pet away to another home. Following the removal of the pet from the house, it is very important that the carpeting be removed and replaced, all upholstered furniture professionally cleaned, and the walls repainted. This aggressive approach can successfully reduce airborne pet allergen to extremely low levels very quickly.

25. How do I know if I need to use an air filter in my house?

Air filters for home use can be divided into those that filter the air, called HEPA filters, and **electrostatic air filters**.

Electrostatic air filter

A filter that places a negative ionic charge upon airborne particles, which then aggregate onto a metal plate in the filter.

HEPA filters consist of a filter and carbon prefilter, which together are capable of filtering particles as small as 0.2 micrometers from room air. HEPA filters will effectively remove both airborne allergens, including molds, animal danders, and pollens, as well as other particles, such as volatile organic compounds and smoke.

As noted in Question 22, house dust mite allergens do not remain airborne for more than a few minutes after being disturbed and are therefore not accessible to air filters.

Electrostatic filters are designed to place a negative ionic charge upon airborne particles, which then aggregate onto a metal plate in the filter. This technology has proven appealing because these filtration devices are small and noiseless. However, they have not proven effective in removing allergens or other particles. In addition, the ozone generated by these machines has proven to be irritating to the respiratory tracts of patients with asthma.

26. Are some dogs truly "hypoallergenic?"

Forty percent of households in the United States own at least one dog and 60% of people have regular contact with a dog either in their own home or in another location. As 10 to 15% of Americans are allergic to dogs, it makes sense that millions of people in this country will have recurring allergic reactions to dogs. The significant allergens are proteins found in the dog's dander (scales sloughed from the dog's skin) and saliva. Differences in allergen production both between breeds and even between individual dogs within a breed may allow people to tolerate some dogs better than others. People's ability to tolerate a specific breed or specific dog is highly variable and not possible to predict given our current knowledge. Some dog breeds have been touted as being "hypoallergenic," suggesting that they are less likely to cause an allergic reaction in people who have been diagnosed as allergic to dogs. These dogs have been characterized as shedding less hair and dander than other dogs, and include but are not limited to poodles, terriers, maltese, schnauzers, and bichon frises, as well as mixes of these breeds with other dogs. While these "low-shedding" dogs may have less obvious shedding of hair, they still shed to some degree, and are capable of causing allergic responses in some people, particularly those who are highly allergic. The amount of the allergen coming from a dog can be reduced or eliminated by bathing the dog once to twice weekly.

27. In what situations will antihistamines be helpful to me?

Antihistamine

An agent that binds to the histamine receptor and blocks the effects of histamine on the body.

Oral **antihistamines** have been in use since the 1950s and play a major role in treating allergic rhinitis. This class of drugs blocks the histamine H_1 receptor. They are most effective in reducing symptoms of sneezing, nasal and ocular itching, and nasal discharge. However, they have very little effect upon nasal congestion. These medications are to be distinguished from histamine H_2 receptor blockers, such as ranitidine and cimetidine, which are largely used to treat gastroesophageal reflux disease and peptic ulcers. Because H_1 antihistamines must bind to the histamine receptor before histamine does, these drugs are most effective when used before coming into contact with a known allergen.

Patients are often concerned that these medications will stop being effective after several weeks or months of use; however, long-term controlled studies have shown that this is not the case. The older antihistamines, including chlorpheniramine, diphenhydramine, and clemastine, are usually taken two to three times per day and are available either alone or in combination with an oral decongestant such as pseudoephedrine. Unfortunately, these older medications pass readily through a membrane around the brain called the "blood–brain barrier" and into the central nervous system, causing sedation in adults and occasionally paradoxic stimulation in children. In addition, these older drugs do not specifically block histamine receptors but also block a number of other chemical receptors, most notably the cholinergic receptors. Blockage of these cholinergic receptors throughout the body often leads to constipation and dryness of the mouth and eyes, and may provoke aggravations of urinary blockage and glaucoma in the elderly.

There is a growing group of newer oral antihistamines, including loratadine, fexofenadine, cetirizine, desloratadine, and levocetirizine (see Table 4 in Question 21). These drugs have onsets of action within 1 to 2 hours and are all taken once daily. Loratadine and cetirizine are now available over the counter in both generic and proprietary formulations These newer antihistamines do not pass as readily through the blood–brain barrier and do not bind to the cholinergic receptors; for these reasons, they cause minimal or no sedation, constipation, or other effects noted with the older antihistamines. Many controlled studies have demonstrated that these medications are equally effective as the older agents. Antihistamines are also available as topical nasal sprays. Both azelastine and olopatadine have been shown to be at least as effective as oral antihistamines and begin to reduce symptoms as quickly as 10 minutes after administration.

28. When do I need a decongestant, and what are the main side effects?

Decongestants, such as pseudoephedrine, act by constricting blood vessels in the nasal membranes and thereby reduce nasal swelling. These drugs have been shown to

Decongestant

An agent that decreases nasal congestion by constricting blood vessels in the nose.

effectively reduce the sensation of nasal congestion but have minimal effects upon other nasal symptoms, such as sneezing, itching of the eyes or nose, or discharge. When given orally, these drugs begin to work within 1 to 2 hours and, depending upon the preparation, may last between 4 and 24 hours. Oral decongestants may have significant side effects, including effects on the brain (insomnia, anxiety, irritability), effects on the cardiovascular system (rapid heartbeat, palpitations, increased blood pressure), and urinary retention, particularly in men with prostatic enlargement.

Oral pseudoephedrine has historically been available over the counter (OTC). Recently, however, OTC use of this medication has become severely restricted—not because of any newly discovered safety issues but because this compound can be chemically converted into methamphetamine.

Nasal decongestant sprays, such as oxymetazoline, act much more quickly than the oral formulations, often within 5 minutes. Because the spray form of these drugs is given in extremely small quantities, there are usually no systemic effects, although very young and much older patients may occasionally have some of the systemic effects previously listed. In addition, when given for longer than 3 to 5 days, patients may experience rebound nasal swelling after stopping the drug, a condition referred to as "rhinitis medicamentosa" (see Question 13).

29. I understand that montelukast is used to treat asthma. Does it help my nasal allergies as well?

Montelukast (Singulair) blocks a chemical called "leukotriene D_4," which causes bronchial spasm and mucus secretion in the lungs and mucosal swelling and mucus secretion in the nose. Montelukast was approved several years ago for the treatment of bronchial asthma in children and adults, and more recently for children and adult patients with seasonal and year-round nasal allergies. While in theory the medication would be expected to work best for nasal congestion and discharge, it has been shown to reduce all nasal symptoms, including sneezing and itching. Clinical trials have demonstrated that montelukast is comparable in effect to oral antihistamines such as loratadine. Montelukast is taken once daily at a dose of 4 mg in children younger than 2 years of age, 5 mg for children between 3 and 14 years, and 10 mg in adolescents older than 14 years and in adults. The side effect profile of this drug has been quite favorable, without any central nervous system side effects such as sedation or anxiety. Recently, the FDA reviewed postmarketing surveillance data that revealed a possible link between montelukast and an increase in suicidal behavior in children. However, careful analysis of all available data from clinical studies does not confirm these findings. Montelukast is best suited for patients with mild rhinitis and can be taken on either a regular or an as-needed basis. Montelukast provides an alternative to oral antihistamines in patients who either do not tolerate antihistamines or whose symptoms are not effectively relieved by these drugs. Some patients with allergic rhinitis may also benefit from a combination of montelukast plus an oral antihistamine, as the two drugs block different chemicals (i.e., histamine and leukotriene D_4) and their clinical effects may be additive. Montelukast should also be considered in patients who have mild persistent asthma along with their allergic rhinitis; in these patients, montelukast may provide satisfactory relief of both upper and lower airway symptoms.

Montelukast provides an alternative to oral antihistamines in patients who either do not tolerate antihistamines or whose symptoms are not effectively relieved by these drugs.

30. Are nasal steroids a useful treatment for nasal allergies?

Steroid medications can be divided into those that are derived from testosterone (androgenic steroids) and those that are related to cortisol (glucocorticoids). Androgenic steroids increase the synthesis of muscle tissue and have minimal effects upon inflammation, while glucocorticoids suppress inflammation and lead to the breakdown of muscle and fat tissue.

Systemically administered glucocorticoids, given orally or by injection, have been used since the 1950s to successfully treat inflammatory diseases such as asthma and arthritis. However, even short-term use of these systemic medications, such as prednisolone (Prednisone), leads to significant systemic side effects, including water and salt retention, increased blood pressure, increased blood sugar, cataracts, increased intraocular pressure, reduced bone mineral density, and mood swings. These adverse effects limit the use of systemic glucocorticoids to patients with very severe disease manifestations. In the 1970s, pharmaceutical companies developed topical intranasal formulations of glucocorticoids to treat allergic rhinitis. In this way, the medication was administered directly to the area of tissue inflammation without causing any systemic effects.

There are a number of intranasal steroids available to treat seasonal and year-round allergic rhinitis in children and adults (**Table 5**), and overall these drugs are the most effective known drug therapy for this disease. Nasal steroids are usually started in patients who have moderate to severe persistent allergic rhinitis. These drugs reduce all symptoms of both seasonal as well as year-round rhinitis, including nasal congestion, nasal itching,

Table 5   Commonly Used Intranasal Steroids (Generic/Brand Name)

Budesonide/Rhinocort Aqua

Fluticasone propionate/Flonase

Mometasone furoate/Nasonex

Triamcinolone acetonide/Nasacort Aq

Ciclesonide/Omnaris

Fluticasone furoate/Veramyst

Flunisolide/Nasarel

sneezing, and discharge. In addition, recent studies show that these medications also reduce symptoms of eye itching and watering.

Jack's comment:

When my allergies started 3 years ago, when I was 28 years old, most of my problems were at night. I was so stuffy that I couldn't sleep, and I had a bad postnasal drip. I tried some Allovert that I got over the counter, but it didn't really change the stuffiness. Then I tried a few doses of Benadryl, and it made me feel sleepy most of the day without really getting rid of the feeling of nasal blockage. Not only that, but it seemed to really dry me out and made me feel constipated. I finally broke down and saw a doctor, and he gave me a sample of Nasonex. After 2 days, I could start to breathe again, and by 1 week I was pretty much back to normal. That medicine made a huge difference in my nasal problem.

31. Are nasal steroids safe for me to take?

The most common adverse effects of intranasal steroids consist of local irritation, with burning and stinging of the nasal mucosa. Approximately 5–10% of patients using these drugs for 2 weeks or longer experience some degree of nasal bleeding, usually consisting of flecks of blood that are seen after forceful blowing of the nose. This problem can be stopped by taking a 3- to 5-day break from the intranasal steroid spray plus the use of a nasal moisturizer before restarting the medication at a lower dose. Systemic effects with an intranasal steroid are quite rare. These medications have been carefully studied in order to determine whether they have any suppressive effects on the function of the adrenal glands; these studies have universally shown no effects. In children, the concern of greatest theoretic importance is suppression of growth. One-year studies with mometasone furoate, fluticasone propionate, and budesonide have failed to show any loss of growth in children between 3 and 11 years of age. In adults, epidemiologic surveys performed to assess the effects of an intranasal steroid on the eyes, including glaucoma and cataracts, have also shown no effects. Taken together, intranasal steroids as a class appear to be extremely safe and have little potential for systemic side effects.

Taken together, intranasal steroids as a class appear to be extremely safe and have little potential for systemic side effects.

32. What is the correct way to use my nasal spray?

There are a number of pointers that may be useful to patients using intranasal sprays. It is important to realize that all available intranasal medications are atomizers that contain a liquid suspension. These types of devices work best when they are held upright in the vertical position and do not spray effectively when they are tilted at an angle or horizontal. Second, all sprays should be directed toward the lateral wall of the nose, which is where most of the nasal swelling is. Instillation of anti-inflammatory sprays, such as intranasal steroids and intranasal antihistamines, directly into this area puts the therapy where it is needed most. Conversely, intranasal steroids should never be sprayed at the middle of the nose where the nasal septum is. The septum has a poor blood supply, and administration of gluco-corticoids toward this area will cause the blood vessels to clamp down, leading to excessive dryness and ultimately nose bleeds. After administering an intranasal steroid, patients should sniff lightly, tilt the head backward, and rock it from side to side. In this way, the medication is allowed to disperse widely and to reach the upper recesses of the nose. When administering intranasal azelastine, however, the patient should instead look toward the floor, head down, for at least 10 seconds after spraying and should not sniff the medication. After lifting his or her head, the patient wipes any excess medication from the nose. This method of delivery helps in reducing the bitter aftertaste associated with azelastine in some patients.

33. Are eye symptoms commonly found in patients with nasal allergies, and how should I treat them?

Approximately 50% of people with nasal allergies also have allergic eye symptoms, known as **allergic conjunctivitis**. The most common symptoms are some combination of redness, itching, and watering. If your eye symptoms are moderately severe and you have not had them before, you should always be checked by a physician to ensure that you do not have an infection or some other eye condition.

Patients often obtain initial treatment of allergic eye symptoms with over-the-counter medications, including oral antihistamines and eyedrops. Oral antihistamines, discussed in Question 27, are moderately effective for eye itching and discharge. Most over-the-counter allergy eyedrops contain topical vasoconstrictors, like

Allergic conjunctivitis

Inflammation of the conjunctivae of the eye due to an allergic reaction. The conjunctivae is the membrane that covers the front of the eye and extends onto the eyelids.

those found in naphazoline (Visine), which should only be used for a few days at a time. When topical vasoconstrictors are used for more than 1 to 2 weeks, patients may develop habituation to the drops with rebound increases in eye symptoms when they are stopped. Ketotifen (sold over the counter as Zaditor, Alaway, and Zyrtec eyedrops) is a medication that both stops the effects of histamine on the eye and prevents mast cells from releasing histamine into the eye. This medication is quite effective and does not cause any adverse effects with chronic use. If ketotifen is not effective in reducing eye symptoms, consult with a physician.

If over-the-counter anti-allergic eyedrops do not relieve the symptoms of allergic conjunctivitis, your physician may recommend a prescription for eyedrops. There are a large number of prescription drops which have been demonstrated to effectively reduce eye itching, redness and watering, including emedastine (Emadine®), cromolyn (Crolom and generics), nedocromil (Alocril and generics), lodoxamide (Alomide), pemirolast (Alamast), olopatadine (Patanol and Pataday), azelastine (Optivar), epinastine (Elestat), and ketorolac (Acular). Patients with a history of aspirin intolerance (typically hives, wheezing, and/or throat swelling) should not use ketorolac, as it is a member of the nonsteroidal anti-inflammatory family of medications. Occasionally, the above medications do not relieve severe symptoms of allergic conjunctivitis and steroid eyedrops are needed for a short (7 to 10 day) period of treatment. Loteprednol (Alrex) is a topical steroid for the eye which is approved for the short-term treatment of allergic conjunctivitis. It must be kept in mind that steroid eyedrops can lead to severe complications, including eye infections, cataracts, and glaucoma, if not used with caution under the close supervision of a physician.

34. I have severe asthma and nasal allergies, and my doctor has prescribed Xolair. Will this help my nasal symptoms as well?

Injectable omalizumab (Xolair) is a relatively new medication that has been approved for use in year-round allergic asthma. This medication, which consists of an antibody against IgE, is injected once to twice per month. Because of its high cost, it is generally reserved for the patients with the most severe allergic asthma. After a few months of treatment, attacks of asthma become significantly less frequent, the need for asthma medications goes down, and patients' quality of life is enhanced. Along with all of these improvements in asthma, nasal symptoms have also been shown to significantly improve. When the drug was given to patients with seasonal hay fever, their allergic nasal and eye symptoms decreased quickly and stayed low while the patients were treated with the drug. Similarly, in patients with year-round allergies caused by dust mites and animal danders, symptoms became much better after a couple of weeks, and the need for oral antihistamines went down. Therefore, if a patient suffers from both asthma and allergic rhinitis, Xolair can be helpful.

35. What are allergy shots, and how effective are they for nasal allergies?

Administration of allergy shots, more appropriately called "specific allergen immunotherapy" or "allergen vaccine therapy," is one of the oldest forms of treatment for allergic rhinitis and conjunctivitis. At the turn of the 20th century, it was discovered that injection of increasing doses of grass allergen into patients with summer hay fever resulted in a marked improvement in seasonal nasal and eye symptoms. It is now recognized that injections of allergenic extracts, including grass, tree, and weed pollens, house dust mites, cat and dog danders, cockroaches, and molds, substantially reduce symptoms of seasonal or perennial rhinitis in up to 80% of patients.

Allergy immunotherapy is usually considered in patients who (1) do not respond adequately to a trial of medications; (2) have significant side effects with medications; (3) begin to develop the involvement of other parts of the respiratory tract in their allergic disease, such as asthma, sinusitis, or middle ear disease; and (4) require a large number of medications that are costly to the patient. Immunotherapy is given once to twice weekly while the dose of allergen is being increased over a period of 4 to 6 months ("build-up phase"). Once the patient has achieved the top dose of allergen extract, the dosing interval is increased to 4 weeks, which is continued for approximately 3 to 4 years ("maintenance phase"), depending upon the response of the patient. Clinical benefits may be seen as soon as 3 months after starting injections but may not become apparent until the patient has been on a full maintenance dose for at least 3 months (usually 9 to 12 months of immunotherapy). Most long-term studies show that the average level of improvement is 50% compared with the baseline level and that this benefit will last at least 2 to 3 years after stopping the therapy. Many patients will have very long-lasting changes in their allergy symptoms, while some will need to restart their shots within 1 year of discontinuing immunotherapy.

The most common adverse effects of allergy vaccine therapy is a large local area of redness, warmth, and itching of the skin at the injection site, which occurs within minutes to hours after the shot. This reaction occurs in at least 10% of patients at some time in their allergy shot program and rarely prevents a patient from reaching the full maintenance dose of allergenic extract. Immediate treatment of the reaction includes the use of ice and oral antihistamines. If these local reactions become recurrent and troublesome, administration of an oral H_1 antihistamine, such as cetirizine (10 mg) or loratadine (10 mg), 2 hours before the shot may be helpful. If this alone does not work, the doctor can add the H_2 antihistamine ranitidine (150 mg) or the leukotriene blocker montelukast (10 mg) , which may provide an additional benefit.

Much more worrisome than these large local skin reactions is the possibility of systemic reactions. These reactions usually occur within 20 to 30 minutes after the injection, and mild systemic reactions may include hives, flushing and itching of the skin, and discharge from the nose. More severe episodes usually involve wheezing, throat swelling, and/or a drop in blood pressure. These more severe reactions are referred to as anaphylaxis, and episodes accompanied by significant drops in blood pressure (<90/60 mm Hg) are referred to as anaphylactic shock. Surveys of large allergy shot populations have shown that approximately 1 in every 200 injections will result in some type of systemic reaction; thus most patients receiving allergy shots will never experience a reaction of this type. Contraindications for starting allergy shots include pregnancy, ischemic heart disease, poorly controlled asthma, and active autoimmune disease, such as systemic lupus erythematosus.

Sarah's comment:

Starting about 5 or 6 years ago, my allergies were so bad that I missed at least a week of school every fall and occasionally in the spring. First, I would have a few days of sneezing and a stuffy, drippy nose, and then the wheezing would kick in, which kept me up half the night two or three nights per week. I used all kinds of antihistamines, nasal sprays, and an inhaler called Advair, which did seem to help a lot. I also used my Proventil inhaler some days up to 5 or 6 times, and I would always end up on a Medrol Dosepak at some point in the fall. My doctor referred me to an allergist, who allergy tested me and found that I was very allergic to birch tree, ragweed, sage weed, and a mold called Alternaria. *He strongly suggested that I take a course of allergy shots, which I have been doing for the past 3 years. After about a year of weekly injections, I began to feel much better, and last spring and fall I only had mild allergies without any major wheezing. I still use my Proventil inhaler but only need it every few days. The shots made a major difference in my life.*

36. Will acupuncture help my nasal allergies?

Acupuncture

The practice of inserting fine needles through the skin at specific points to treat disease or relieve pain.

Acupuncture is an ancient form of therapy that originated in Asia and is now practiced throughout the world for a large number of physical illnesses. In the United States, approximately 2 million people, or close to 1% of the population, seek acupuncture care each year, and 4% of the US population have used acupuncture at some time in their lives. There have been over 100 clinical studies that have examined whether acupuncture treatment is helpful in reducing the symptoms of allergic rhinitis. The results of a thorough analysis of all relevant data concluded that for seasonal allergic rhinitis, acupuncture had no detectable beneficial effects. However, for year-round chronic symptoms of nasal allergy, there was an overall improvement in nasal symptoms, and in some studies this effect was stronger than allergy medications. None of these studies were designed to determine whether acupuncture induced a long-lasting "cure" of nasal allergy.

The safety of acupuncture has been examined carefully, and in general, the rate of adverse events is quite low. In infants, acupuncture should be avoided in areas on top of the head until the fontanel (open spot in the skull bone) is closed. Studies have determined that in children, there is an approximate 1–2% risk of an adverse event and serious reactions are rare (1 in 10,000 children).

In a small number of my patients, conventional allergy treatments (medications and/or allergy shots) have not adequately relieved the patient's symptoms. In patients who are inclined, I would not dissuade them from a trial of acupuncture, keeping in mind that they will require regular visits to a practitioner for a long period of time with no evidence that a persistent remission will be achieved.

37. Which herbal products will help my nasal allergies?

Herbal remedies have a long track record of use throughout much of the world for a variety of ailments and have become increasingly popular in the United States over the past 2 decades. Patients are often attracted to the fact that these products are found in nature and that they have been used by indigenous cultures around the world for very long periods of time. There is also a generalized concept that because they are "natural," they are safer. It is important to keep in mind, however, that these substances may also cause significant side effects.

A number of herbs have been used to treat symptoms of allergic rhinitis. Botanical products that have been tested in clinical trials and demonstrated improvement in allergic rhinitis symptoms include butterbur root, stinging nettle, and tomato seed extract. Another large group of plant-derived substances, including *Citrus unshiu,*

Lycopus lucidus plant, *Amomum xanthiodes* plant, a Chinese herbal medication (bu-zhong-yi-qi-tang), and spirulina algae, have been shown to have beneficial anti-allergic effects in laboratory experiments but have not been tested in patients with allergic rhinitis. Grape seed extract has not been shown to have any significant effects in allergic rhinitis.

38. When should I take my child to an allergy specialist?

If your child develops symptoms of seasonal nasal allergies, his or her physician will prescribe medications, such as oral antihistamines or intranasal steroids, for the symptoms. If these medications are effective, and do not result in any unwanted side effects, they can be used safely on a seasonal basis for many years. Because seasonal nasal symptoms are almost always related to an outdoor pollen or mold, there is no need to do allergy testing unless your child stops responding to the medications or develops side effects. At that point, if your child is 5 years of age or older, he or she should be referred to an allergist for allergy testing in order to precisely identify which seasonal allergens are causing the symptoms in preparation for allergy immunotherapy. Allergy testing to foods should only be included if the child also has symptoms directly related to eating.

If your child has year-round nasal symptoms particularly if they are older than 2 years of age, allergy testing should be performed in order to confirm a diagnosis of allergic rhinitis and determine whether there is an allergen that can be actively avoided. The patient's environmental history will guide the testing; for example, the doctor will ascertain whether there is a pet in the house. The allergens most often included are house dust mites, animal danders, cockroaches, and both indoor and outdoor molds. This initial testing need not be extensive and can be performed as either an allergy skin or blood test. Some primary care physicians are comfortable in performing a screening allergy blood test and are prepared to make recommendations regarding allergen avoidance based upon these results. If the primary care doctor is not inclined toward ordering the appropriate blood tests or devising programs of environmental control, your child may be referred to an allergist at this point.

Other situations in which your child should be referred to an allergist include the development of other related diseases, particularly bronchial asthma, recurrent or chronic sinusitis, or recurrent or persistent middle ear disease in association with their rhinitis. In addition, another concern is the development of oral abnormalities caused by chronic mouth breathing.

39. Do nasal allergies worsen during pregnancy, and how should they be treated?

Women go through a number of important physiologic and immunologic changes during pregnancy. Blood volume and estrogen levels both increase during pregnancy, which frequently lead to mucous membrane swelling in the nose. For this reason, many women who have no history of rhinitis develop nasal congestion during pregnancy. Women with allergic rhinitis may develop worsening nasal symptoms while pregnant, although it has been estimated that roughly equal numbers of women experience an increase, reduction, or no change in their nasal allergic symptoms. In my own experience, the majority of women develop worsening symptoms while pregnant, usually consisting of nasal congestion.

Many women who have no history of rhinitis develop nasal congestion during pregnancy.

Treatment of allergic rhinitis during pregnancy must always consider the effect of the therapy upon the growing fetus. Given the capacity of many medications to have potential effects upon fetal development, it is critical to determine what the woman is allergic to in order to set up a program of allergen avoidance measures. If the patient has not been previously allergy tested, I counsel against performing allergy skin testing because of the small but possible risk of a systemic reaction. Rather, it is preferable to do blood tests, which can serve as a sound basis for environmental control measures for house dust mites, animal danders, molds, and pollens.

Despite avoiding relevant allergens, most women with significant nasal allergies will require some medication to successfully treat their symptoms. The FDA has created a rating system that classifies all medicines approved since 1980 into five categories (**Table 6**), referred to as A, B, C, D, and X. Category A is considered the safest, while category X medications are absolutely contraindicated under any circumstances. None of the medications used for allergic rhinitis are classified as category A, and the majority of drugs used for rhinitis fall into categories B and C. We always try to start with category B drugs, adding any required medications that are labeled category C. Keeping safety in mind, medications should be directed at specific symptoms. If sneezing, nasal discharge, and itching of the eyes and nose are the predominant symptoms, either intranasal cromolyn spray or oral antihistamines may be adequate. Nasal cromolyn, which is available over the counter, is not absorbed to any significant degree into the bloodstream and is therefore considered one of the safest allergy medications to take during pregnancy. Loratadine and cetirizine are

Table 6   FDA Drug Ratings for Use in Pregnancy

Category	Interpretation
A	Adequate, well-controlled studies in pregnant women have not shown an increased risk of fetal abnormalities to the fetus in any trimester of pregnancy.
B	Animal studies have revealed no evidence of harm to the fetus; however, there are no adequate and well-controlled studies in pregnant women. OR Animal studies have shown an adverse effect, but adequate and well-controlled studies in pregnant women have failed to demonstrate a risk to the fetus in any trimester.
C	Animal studies have shown an adverse effect and there are no adequate and well-controlled studies in pregnant women. OR No animal studies have been conducted and there are no adequate and well-controlled studies in pregnant women.
D	Adequate well-controlled or observational studies in pregnant women have demonstrated a risk to the fetus. However, the benefits of therapy may outweigh the potential risk. For example, the drug may be acceptable if needed in a life-threatening situation or serious disease for which safer drugs cannot be used or are ineffective.
X	Adequate well-controlled or observational studies in animals or pregnant women have demonstrated positive evidence of fetal abnormalities or risks. The use of the product is contraindicated in women who are or may become pregnant.

both category B medications, and loratadine is usually favored due to its longer record of use in pregnancy. Diphenhydramine and chlorpheniramine are older drugs that have been used extensively in pregnancy. However, both of these drugs cause significant sleepiness and fatigue and are not tolerated well by many patients. If nasal congestion presents as the most prominent symptom, as it often does during pregnancy, nasal steroids are indicated. Budesonide (Rhinocort Aqua) is rated as category B, while other intranasal steroids, including ciclesonide, fluticasone propionate, mometasone furoate, and triamcinolone acetonide, are category C. Other drugs that are effective for nasal congestion include pseudo-ephedrine, which should be avoided during the first trimester because of an increased risk of infantile gastroschisis (herniation of intestines outside of the body).

If you become pregnant while taking allergy shots, the shots can be continued at whatever dose is currently being given and should not be increased until after the baby is delivered because of concerns regarding systemic reactions. For this same reason, allergy shots should not be initiated during pregnancy. If you are pregnant and have questions regarding allergy shots and allergy medications, you should consult with your treating physicians. Your obstetrician, primary care doctor, and possibly a consulting allergist may all provide guidance regarding these treatment issues. It is best not to stop or alter your treatment regimen unless you have discussed potential changes with them.

Jacquelyn's comment:

I had really mild allergies for most of my life, and when I became pregnant, things changed quickly. The first thing I noticed was that I couldn't breathe through my nose at night because of stuffiness, and then I started to have a postnasal drip that wouldn't go away. My ob-gyn doctor gave me Benadryl to take at night. It made the drip really thick, and my nose was still quite blocked up. Besides that, I was so sleepy that I couldn't get up in the morning. I got Claritin after that, which didn't make me sleepy but wasn't any more effective than the Benadryl. I saw an allergist, who prescribed Rhinocort twice a day, and after a few days my nose finally opened up enough so I could sleep at night. He assured me that it was safe during pregnancy.

40. Will I be able to breast-feed my child while I am taking allergy medications?

The medications listed in Question 39 can all be used while you are breast-feeding your baby. However, most of these medications will pass from the bloodstream into the breast milk and cause similar systemic side effects as those seen in the mother. Therefore, older, sedating antihistamines such as diphenhydramine and chlorpheniramine may also result in significant sedation in the nursing infant. Topical medications, such as intranasal steroids and intranasal antihistamines, are not typically well absorbed into the bloodstream and will therefore have minimal effects on the baby.

41. When I fly, my nasal allergies get worse. What can I do to prevent this?

The two biggest factors that cause allergy sufferers to experience problems on planes is the change in cabin pressure, particularly during descent, and the low humidity of the cabin. The change in pressure often leads to swelling of the sinus openings, with subsequent sinus headaches, and closure of the eustachian tubes, with secondary ear pain or even bleeding into the middle ear (middle ear hemorrhage). The best method for preventing these symptoms is the use of an over-the-counter topical decongestant, such as oxymetazoline, 30 to 60 minutes before the plane begins its descent. Taking your daily allergy medications before, during, and after the flight, according to your usual schedule, is also helpful.

Low cabin humidity, which is normal during flights, leads to increased dryness of the nasal mucous membranes, which may further aggravate nasal, sinus, and eustachian tube swelling. To help counteract this problem, a saline nasal spray every 2 hours during the flight

Topical medications, such as intranasal steroids and intranasal antihistamines, are not typically well absorbed into the bloodstream and will therefore have minimal effects on the baby.

47

can help. In addition, increased oral intake of fluids may also be useful. Alcoholic beverages, which are known to increase urination, may reduce your state of hydration and are therefore best avoided on plane trips by individuals with nasal allergies or sinus problems.

42. My 5-year-old daughter has had chronic fluid in both ears. Does she need to be evaluated for allergies?

Otitis media with effusion

Inflammation of the middle ear with resultant fluid collection in the middle ear space.

Acute middle ear infections (acute otitis media) usually follow colds, and occasionally the fluid in the middle ear space persists for long periods of time. Chronic middle ear fluid, referred to as **otitis media with effusion**, is defined as mild middle ear inflammation with fluid but without symptoms of fever, pain, and infection. The most common symptoms of chronic middle ear fluid in infants are irritability or sleep disturbances, failure to respond appropriately to voice or environmental sounds, balance problems, unexplained clumsiness, delayed development of gross motor skills, speech or language, and other signs of hearing loss (such as listening to the television at a very high volume). Common complaints in a 5-year-old child with persistent middle ear fluid would be rubbing of the ears, mild intermittent ear pain, fullness or "popping" of the ears, and problems with school performance. However, in approximately half of children with persistent middle ear fluid, neither the children nor their parents describe significant complaints.

Many factors contribute to the chances that a child will develop chronic middle ear fluid, including the age and genetic background of the child, shape of the middle ear structures, as well as exposure to viral infections, airborne allergens, and irritants (such as tobacco smoke). Many studies have shown that children with nasal allergies are at increased risk for developing chronic middle ear fluid, particularly those older than 3 years of age. While the connection between allergies and middle ear fluid are not completely clear, we do understand that nasal allergy can lead to swelling of the eustachian tubes, which alters the pressure within the middle ear and predisposes the ear space to fluid accumulation.

In children with chronic ear fluid who also have persistent nasal symptoms, it is useful to perform allergy tests. If the tests show positive results, I would counsel the family regarding allergen avoidance measures and prescribe appropriate medical treatment. If these steps do not alleviate the child's allergy symptoms, I would consider prescribing allergy immunotherapy. In the event that a patient has no symptoms of rhinitis, I would not pursue allergy testing; nor would I prescribe anti-allergic treatment.

43. Do allergies increase the need for orthodontia in children?

Children may experience chronic blockage of the nose for a variety of reasons, including allergic rhinitis, non–allergic rhinitis, or enlargement of the adenoid gland. When the child lies down to sleep, the blockage often becomes worse because of increased blood flow through the nasal mucosal tissue due to gravity, which causes the membranes to swell. In addition, the blockage may worsen because of positional factors that cause the adenoid gland to encroach upon the upper airway. When nasal obstruction becomes severe, either during the night or day, the breathing pattern shifts from breathing through the nose to breathing primarily through the mouth, which may result in snoring, dryness of the mouth, and sore throat. In addition, mouth breathing places the oral cavity under significant stress and eventually causes the palate of the mouth to become narrow and high-arched and the lower jaw to move backward toward the neck. These anatomic changes ultimately cause the teeth to become crowded and may lead to the development of an overbite. Oral problems like this are often noticed around age 4 or 5 years; once established, they may require a palatal expander and other orthodontic appliances to enlarge the palate and straighten the teeth. These orofacial problems highlight the importance of diagnosing and treating nasal blockage in young children.

44. What is sinusitis, and how is it related to allergies?

The paranasal sinuses are air-filled cavities located inside the bone of the human skull. While we are not entirely sure of their function, we do know that air pockets within solid structures provide increased strength and reduced weight. The four principal sinuses include the maxillary sinuses (in the cheeks), the frontal sinuses (in the forehead), the anterior and posterior ethmoid sinuses (which are a collection of very small cavities between the eyes), and the sphenoid sinuses (behind the nose and under the brain) (**Figure 2**). Sinusitis is a

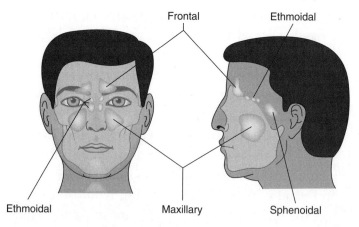

Figure 2   Location of the paranasal sinuses.

condition characterized by inflammation of the mucosal lining of one or more of these sinuses.

Acute sinusitis is a bacterial infection of the paranasal sinuses that follows a typical cold. While colds usually resolve within 5 to 7 days, patients with acute sinusitis usually have symptoms of worsening facial pain and yellow or green nasal discharge. Acute sinusitis is usually diagnosed on clinical grounds, and x-rays are generally not needed.

Chronic sinusitis is most often suspected when patients have had some combination of upper airway symptoms including discolored postnasal drip, nasal congestion, facial fullness or headache, cough, and/or sore throat for longer than 3 months. The pathogenesis of chronic sinusitis is not entirely understood, but there is increasing evidence to support the idea that allergies can predispose a person to persistent sinus inflammation. Allergies do this by causing swelling of the areas where the sinuses drain into the nose, preventing secretions from leaving the sinuses. Very much like allergic rhinitis, nonallergic rhinitis can do the same thing, inducing persistent inflammation of the drainage tracts of the sinuses.

Other causes of recurrent sinus infections include structural abnormalities within the nasal passages and sinuses, such as a deviated septum (the structure that divides the nasal passage into two sides) and other bony abnormalities that may prevent the sinuses from draining. These abnormalities are usually found with CT (computed tomography) scans of the sinuses, and they may require surgery. Many patients have acid reflux, which in severe cases may go all the way up to the throat and nose and result in persistent inflammation. Problems with low

Acute sinusitis

Inflammation of the mucosal lining of the paranasal sinuses lasting more than 10 days and usually associated with bacterial infection. Antibiotics are generally required for resolution of symptoms.

Chronic sinusitis

Inflammation of the mucosal lining of the paranasal sinuses that persists for more than 3 months.

51

immune function, particularly involving the formation of antibodies, can predispose people to various types of infections, including sinusitis. Rarely, cystic fibrosis, which causes a genetic abnormality in mucus thickness, and primary ciliary problems, which result in an inability to clear secretions, may cause chronic sinus problems.

45. How should chronic sinus problems be treated?

A general approach to patients with chronic sinusitis includes nasal saline flushes, intranasal steroids, and a prolonged course (at least 3 weeks) of a broad-spectrum antibiotic (**Table 7**). In approximately half of patients with chronic sinusitis, patients are found to have positive skin tests to airborne allergens. Given this very high prevalence of allergy in chronic sinusitis, it seems worthwhile to do allergy testing in all patients with this condition. If the results show that the patient is allergic to an avoidable allergen, particularly a year-around allergen such as house dust mites, indoor pets, and indoor mold, aggressive allergen avoidance measures should be started promptly. A small number of clinical studies suggest that allergy vaccine therapy (allergy shots) may be helpful in reducing the severity of chronic sinusitis, and most physicians will start a trial of this treatment in patients with relevant positive skin tests. If this initial program of allergen avoidance, medications, and possibly immunotherapy is not successful after a several-week trial,

Table 7 Overall Treatment Approach to Chronic Sinusitis

Nasal irrigation
Intranasal steroids
Oral antibiotics
Allergen avoidance and immunotherapy (if allergic)

endoscopic sinus surgery may be employed to remove diseased mucosal tissue, particularly from the very narrow drainage tracts that empty from the sinuses into the nose.

Endoscopy

Examination of the body's interior through an instrument inserted into a natural opening or an incision.

Susan's comment:

I've had allergies most of my life. When I was a child, it was mostly during the spring and summer months. As I got older, the symptoms seemed to stretch out through the whole year, mostly with a stuffy nose and a drip in my throat. Over the last 2 years, I've been having sinus infections, where the mucus turns green and I have a bad cough and headache. This happens every 2 or 3 months, and I have to get an antibiotic from my doctor. For the past 6 months, I've been taking a nasal spray called Veramyst every day. I still have some nasal congestion, but the repeated infections have become less frequent, and overall I feel much better.

46. What are nasal polyps, and are they caused by allergies?

Nasal polyps are teardrop-shaped growths that usually start in the sinus cavity and extend into the nose. There is no relationship between nasal polyps and polyps in the colon. Small nasal polyps often cause no symptoms and go unnoticed, while larger ones can completely block the nasal passages. Although their origin is not really known, they most often begin in patients who have chronically inflamed sinuses. We do know that somewhere between 30% and 50% of patients with nasal polyps have positive skin tests to allergens, indicating that allergy may be a contributing cause in a large subset of patients. Nasal polyps are more likely to occur in adults, patients with asthma, patients with allergic-like reactions to aspirin and other nonsteroidal anti-inflammatory drugs (e.g., ibuprofen), and people with a family history of nasal polyps. Polyps are extremely

Nasal polyp

A growth that usually originates in the mucous membrane of the sinus cavity and extends into the nose.

uncommon in children unless cystic fibrosis is present. The most common symptoms of nasal polyps are nasal discharge (often thick in consistency and yellow in color), nasal stuffiness, loss of taste and smell, postnasal drip, facial pain, and snoring. Of all these symptoms, the one that is most suggestive that polyps are present is the reduction in taste and smell.

Diagnosis of nasal polyps is usually made when your physician can see the polyp during a routine nasal examination. However, once polyps are suspected, more in-depth examinations will often be made, including nasal endoscopy (by an otolaryngologist or allergist) or CT scanning of the sinuses. When polyps are left untreated, they place patients at risk for frequent sinus infections, obstructive sleep apnea, and, in the most severe cases, changes in facial structure (such as a widening of the bridge of the nose). Treatment of nasal polyps almost always includes intranasal steroids. This treatment may shrink the polyps or eliminate them completely. However, if a nasal corticosteroid is not effective, your doctor may prescribe a short (5 to 10 days) course of an oral corticosteroid, such as prednisone, either alone or in combination with an intranasal steroid spray. Your doctor may also prescribe other drugs to treat conditions that contribute to chronic inflammation in your sinuses or nasal passages, such as antihistamines to treat allergies, antibiotics to treat a chronic or recurring infection, or antifungal medications to treat symptoms of fungal infection.

When polyps are left untreated, they place patients at risk for frequent sinus infections, obstructive sleep apnea, and, in the most severe cases, changes in facial structure (such as a widening of the bridge of the nose).

If drug treatment does not shrink or eliminate your nasal polyps, your doctor may recommend surgery. The type of surgery depends on the size, number, and location of the polyps. For small polyps, many physicians will opt to perform a polypectomy (excision of the polyp), which is usually an office procedure. For more extensive cases, particularly when there is a large amount of chronic sinus inflammation, endoscopic sinus surgery may be recommended. After surgery, you will likely use an intranasal steroid to help prevent the recurrence of nasal polyps. In addition, if you have significant allergies, allergy vaccine treatment may be beneficial in controlling the concomitant symptoms of allergy.

47. Can chronic headaches be related to allergies?

Headaches may be related to allergic rhinitis in a number of ways. First, patients with severe nasal congestion may have swelling of the openings to the paranasal sinuses, called "ostia." This swelling may cause intermittent or persistent closure of the sinus, resulting in an inability to equalize pressure within the sinus cavity. Symptoms related to sinus pressure include pain or pressure over the forehead, between the eyes, or over the cheeks, brought on or aggravated by changes in barometric pressure (flying, driving into the mountains, or during weather changes) or while bending forward. These headaches often respond to medications that effectively reduce nasal swelling, such as intranasal steroids. Second, many patients with allergic rhinitis have some degree of concomitant chronic sinusitis. In these cases, the sinuses may be persistently blocked or filled with inflammatory tissue and/or active infection. Typically, in these patients, a number of symptoms and signs will be present, such as thick, discolored postnasal drip, sore throat, and/or cough. Third, a significant minority of patients with allergic rhinitis suffer from migraine headaches, which may be triggered or aggravated by nasal swelling. In addition, some patients with allergic rhinitis may also suffer from food allergies, which may provoke migraines. Finally, some patients who use intranasal medications complain that putting any type of nasal spray into their nose directly triggers a headache. Each of these various mechanisms should be considered in all patients who suffer from allergic rhinitis and headaches, and patients should be treated accordingly.

48. Do nasal allergies affect bronchial asthma?

A number of long-term studies of large populations have shown that patients who have allergic rhinitis frequently have subtle narrowing and inflammation of the bronchial tubes in the absence of any asthma symptoms. When patients with isolated seasonal or year-around nasal allergies are followed over time, they are found to have an increased risk of developing asthma compared to the general population. In patients who have both allergic rhinitis and asthma, the severity of nasal symptoms and asthma are strongly correlated, and patients with severe rhinitis require significantly more medication to control their asthma.

There are a number of significant benefits that may occur when rhinitis is treated in patients who have nasal allergy and asthma. In patients with seasonal hay fever and allergic asthma, giving a nasal steroid or an oral antihistamine reduces asthma symptoms and causes small but significant improvements in breathing test results. In patients with allergic rhinitis and more severe asthma, taking a nasal steroid reduces the number of major asthma attacks that require treatment in an emergency room or admission to a hospital. In children with exercise-induced asthma, a nasal steroid allows the child to exercise without developing symptoms or signs of asthma. Just as importantly, patients with nasal allergies who do not yet have asthma may benefit from some types of allergy treatment. Allergy shots administered for 2 or more years can significantly reduce the chances of developing asthma. All of these findings make a strong case for treating nasal allergies aggressively in patients with both rhinitis and asthma, and in using allergy shots in allergy patients who have not yet developed asthma.

Roger's comment:

I've had spring allergies for a long time, probably since I was in college. I'm 36 years old now, and over the past couple of years, my hay fever gets so bad that none of the over-the-counter medicines, like Benadryl or Alavert, help that much. Last year, I became more concerned because I noticed wheezing in my chest, especially when my nose was plugged up. This past spring season, the same problem started happening, and I saw a doctor who prescribed Omnaris spray and a pill called Singulair. I was worried that the Omnaris is a steroid, but the doctor explained that steroids sprayed into the nose do not have any significant side effects. The two medications really helped clear up my nose, and I stopped wheezing too.

49. How does nasal allergy affect sleep?

Patients with nasal allergies often have fatigue during the day. One of the main causes of this tiredness is poor sleep quality during the night. Sleep studies of patients with allergic rhinitis have shown that they repeatedly come out of the deepest phases of sleep and enter periods of lighter sleep; these periods of near-awakening are referred to as "micro-arousals." Some patients will experience breaks in their normal breathing pattern, but complete stoppage of breathing (apnea) is unusual. These abnormalities in sleep are most strongly related to the degree of nasal congestion. Medications aimed at relieving nasal congestion, such as intranasal steroids, appear to correct some of these abnormalities in breathing during sleep in patients with allergies.

50. Will moving to a new area help my allergies?

Patients with seasonal or year-round allergies occasionally experience such difficulty with their nasal allergies that they consider moving to another geographic location to help reduce their symptoms. Patients with seasonal hay fever will often find that many of the seasonal pollens and/or molds that bother them in their current home will also be present in areas they are considering moving to. One exception may be ragweed pollen, which is much more commonly seen at high levels east of the Rocky Mountains. With respect to perennial allergens, house dust mites are found in much higher quantities in areas with outdoor relative humidity greater than 45% (particularly near bodies of water), while they tend to be sparse in areas of lower humidity (in deserts and mountains). Therefore, if a patient is primarily allergic to mites, moving to a more arid climate with low levels of dust mites might theoretically improve symptoms. However, other factors, such as air pollution, extremes in outdoor temperature, and the effect of dry air, may also contribute to nasal symptoms in an unpredictable way, thereby making it difficult to categorically recommend a change in location.

51. How is nasal allergy related to mood and energy level?

Many studies have shown that people with allergic rhinitis have problems with mood and energy.

Many studies have shown that people with allergic rhinitis have problems with mood and energy. In a survey of 2500 people with allergies, nearly 1 in 4 people felt embarrassed as a result of their allergy symptoms, more than one-third felt depressed, and over half felt irritable or miserable because of their allergies. In addition, 80% of this group felt tired as a result of their allergy symptoms. The reasons for these findings are not completely understood, but a number of factors may contribute. First, the effects of allergy upon sleep (as discussed in Question 49) can have a significant impact on psychological functioning. Second, we know that multiple different chemicals are elevated in the bloodstream during allergic reactions, which can affect energy and mood. In addition, commonly used allergy medications, particularly older antihistamines (e.g., diphenhydramine) and oral decongestants (e.g., pseudoephedrine), may also cause patients to feel tired, depressed, and/or anxious. It makes sense, therefore, that effective treatment of allergies may improve a person's mood and energy level.

PART THREE

Food Allergy

Can chemicals in food cause allergic reactions?

What is the best test for diagnosing food allergies?

If I am allergic to peanuts, how careful do I have to be?

More . . .

52. How do foods cause adverse reactions?

There are two main ways that a food can cause bothersome physical symptoms. The first category is what we call a food hypersensitivity. These reactions occur when your immune system responds abnormally to proteins in specific foods. These immunologic reactions may be caused by IgE antibodies, which we refer to as a food allergy, or may be related to mechanisms that do not involve IgE. Patients with food allergy due to IgE antibodies often have gastrointestinal symptoms (nausea, vomiting, diarrhea, and abdominal cramping), skin reactions (hives and eczema), and full-blown systemic reactions, also called "anaphylaxis" (throat swelling, wheezing, and drop in blood pressure). Food hypersensitivity that is not related to IgE antibodies includes a number of relatively rare disorders, such as food-induced enterocolitis (inflammation of the colon) and celiac disease (immune reaction to gluten).

The second large category of reactions is referred to as food intolerance reactions. These adverse responses to foods are relatively common and are not related to any immunologic mechanism. A good example is lactose intolerance.

53. Which foods are patients most commonly allergic to?

Peanuts, soybeans, tree nuts, eggs, cow's milk, wheat, shellfish, and fish are the most commonly reported allergenic foods. Allergy to peanuts, soy, tree nuts, eggs, milk, or wheat often develop early in the first few years of life, while hypersensitivity to shellfish or fish more often manifests in adulthood. Allergy to milk or eggs frequently resolves between age 3 and 5 years, while allergy to peanut, tree nuts, shellfish, or fish often lasts through a patient's lifetime.

Nancy's comment:

As a baby, I had a milk and egg allergy with rashes after eating small amounts of these foods. When I was around 4 years old, I ate a peanut butter and jelly sandwich and immediately had an itchy red rash around my mouth. I started seeing an allergist right after that, and allergy skin tests showed that I was allergic to milk, eggs, and peanuts. When I was 6 years old, I was no longer allergic to eggs and milk and was able to start eating them again. I accidentally ate candy with peanuts in it at age 9, and I broke out with hives all over my body. I have been followed by an allergist since then, and I am now 26 years old and am still allergic to peanuts.

54. What is lactose intolerance?

Most reactions to milk, particularly those that occur primarily in the gastrointestinal tract, are not allergic in nature. The most common adverse reaction to milk, which usually starts around age 7 or 8 years, is **lactose intolerance**. Symptoms of lactose intolerance, which include abdominal cramping, gassiness, nausea, and diarrhea, occur between 30 minutes to 2 hours after consuming milk products. Lactose intolerance is caused by an inability to digest significant amounts of lactose, which is the major sugar found in milk. Lactose intolerance is caused by a shortage of the enzyme lactase, which is produced by cells in the small intestine. Some people who are deficient in lactase do not have symptoms of lactose intolerance unless they eat very large amounts of dairy-containing foods.

Lactose intolerance

Inability to digest lactose, which is a principal sugar of milk, which causes symptoms of diarrhea, abdominal pain, and bloating.

Patients who develop lactose intolerance early in life are considered to have a "primary" lactase deficiency. Older patients with chronic digestive diseases, such as ulcerative colitis, may also develop lactose intolerance. These patients are considered to have a "secondary" lactase deficiency.

Up to 15% of all Americans are lactose intolerant, while the figure rises to 80% in African Americans, 80% in Native Americans, and 90% in Asian Americans.

Up to 15% of all Americans are lactose intolerant, while the figure rises to 80% in African Americans, 80% in Native Americans, and 90% in Asian Americans. Premature babies may also be lactose intolerant, as lactase does not increase to full levels until the last trimester of pregnancy.

Lactose intolerance may be difficult to diagnose based on symptoms alone, and the first step often taken by a physician is to eliminate all cow-based dairy products from the diet to see if the symptoms go away. The most common diagnostic test used to confirm questionable cases of lactose intolerance is the hydrogen breath test, which may be ordered by a doctor in confusing cases.

Janet's comment:

I had a really bad stomach infection after a trip to Mexico last summer. I ate food from some small stands, and later that night I had diarrhea and cramps. I was sick for about a week and saw my doctor. She gave me Cipro to take for a few days, and I felt better. After that, I noticed that whenever I ate a lot of cheese or had cereal and milk, I started cramping again and my stools were loose. After a couple of weeks of this, I went back to my doctor, and she suspected that the gastrointestinal infection had caused me to become temporarily lactose intolerant. I've been avoiding all dairy for the past month, without any more stomach symptoms, and my doctor said she believed that, over the next few months, I should go back to normal and be able to have dairy again.

55. How is lactose intolerance treated?

There are no medications or other treatments that increase the amount of lactase enzyme in the intestine. However, gastrointestinal symptoms can be prevented through a special diet. Most people with lactose intolerance do not have to avoid lactose completely, but people differ in the amounts and types of milk-containing foods they can handle. For example, one person may have symptoms after drinking a few sips of milk, while others can drink one glass but not two. Certain foods are better tolerated than others: yogurt is tolerated better than cheese, and cheese better than whole milk. For those people with lactose intolerance who have trouble limiting their intake of dairy-containing foods, the lactase enzyme can be taken as a pill or liquid supplement, which makes lactose more digestible. Lactose-reduced milk and other products are also available at most supermarkets.

56. Can food additives, such as preservatives, cause allergic reactions?

Food additives, including preservatives, flavor enhancers, and artificial colorings and sweeteners, are found in virtually all processed foods. As a general rule, food additives are unusual causes of food-related symptoms. However, in situations in which no food protein can be identified as the cause of a food reaction, additives should be considered.

The additive most commonly implicated in adverse reactions to foods is the family of chemicals called "sulfites." Commercially available as sodium and potassium bisulfite, sodium and potassium metabisulfite, and sulfur dioxide, these agents are used to prevent oxidation of foods, including but not limited to white wine, dried fruit, and dried potatoes. They are also applied to fresh foods, such as vegetables in salad bars, fresh seafood, and peeled potatoes, to prevent discoloration. The most common reaction to eating sulfites is the development of acute wheezing in patients with pre-existing asthma. Rarely, sulfites have been described as causing acute, severe systemic reactions as well.

Food dyes, particularly tartrazine (yellow dye no. 5) has been shown to occasionally aggravate chronic hives. This dye is used frequently in foods, such as hard candy, and may also be added to certain medications, including a variety of medicinal syrups (even those used to treat allergy symptoms!).

Monosodium glutamate (MSG) is a flavor enhancer used in many prepared foods and was once a common ingredient in Chinese restaurants. Beginning in the 1970s, people reported that MSG caused acute, transient symptoms of headache, disorientation, and occasionally chest pain. However, carefully performed clinical studies have failed to conclusively demonstrate any link between MSG and these symptoms. In any event, many restaurants no longer add MSG to their freshly cooked foods, making it easier to avoid this additive.

Butylated hydroxyanisole (BHA) and butylated hydroxytoluene (BHT) are commonly used preservatives that have been suspected of causing hives. However, studies show that these additives are well-tolerated and have not been shown to provoke rashes or any other symptoms.

As mentioned earlier, intolerance of these chemicals should be considered in patients with acute reactions to foods. However, definitive confirmation that food additives are the cause of physical symptoms is usually very difficult. Once it can be established that a particular additive was present in a meal that preceded symptoms, it must next be shown that the additive was a plausible cause of the patient's symptoms. For instance, sodium metabisulfite would be important in a patient with an attack of asthma but might be much less relevant in a patient with headache. Unfortunately, there are no good laboratory evaluations, such as a blood or skin test, to diagnose a sensitivity to these additives. Therefore, the initial diagnosis may be based upon clinical observations that the additive caused specific symptoms on more than one occasion and that these symptoms did not occur when the additive was avoided. Following these observations, an oral challenge with the additive may be considered to confirm the diagnosis. These challenges are time consuming and technically demanding and require special materials; for these reasons, they are performed in specialized centers.

57. Can peanut oil cause allergy symptoms in patients who are allergic to peanuts?

Most cooking oils that are commercially produced, including peanut oil, are highly refined using a hot solvent extraction method, causing the protein to be removed from the product. Since it is the proteins in foods that are responsible for food allergy, these highly refined oils are typically considered nonallergenic. Observations made over many years have demonstrated that people with severe peanut allergy do not have allergic reactions to processed oils. While most large grocery stores and restaurants sell or use oils that are solvent extracted, patients may occasionally encounter cold-pressed oils, which may be marketed as gourmet products. These oils may contain allergenic proteins and should therefore be carefully avoided by all peanut-allergic patients. For the same reason, allergic individuals should avoid oils that have been used to fry potentially allergenic foods.

58. My child is allergic to eggs. Is it safe for her to receive vaccines?

Vaccines for measles, mumps, and rubella (MMR) and influenza are both raised in egg-based cell cultures, prompting concerns about the safety of these vaccines in children who are allergic to eggs. Careful analyses of the MMR vaccine have demonstrated that it does not contain egg proteins capable of causing a reaction in an egg-allergic individual. Based upon a long record of safety, the American Academy of Pediatrics recommends that children with egg allergy be given the MMR vaccine without any special measures being taken. In our own practice, we monitor egg-allergic children in our office for 60 minutes after administration of the MMR vaccine. The influenza vaccine, however, does contain small amounts of egg protein. Patients with true egg allergy can first be skin tested to the influenza vaccine; if they have a negative result, the vaccine can be safely administered as a single dose. If the skin test is positive, the vaccine can still be given, but it should be done by an allergist who can safely give the vaccine in multiple small doses over a few hours while closely monitoring the person for an allergic reaction.

59. If I'm allergic to gelatin, can I receive vaccines?

Gelatin protein, which is found in Jell-O gelatin and pudding desserts, is normally added to many vaccines as a heat stabilizer. Routine childhood vaccines containing gelatin include MMR, varicella (chicken pox), influenza, and DTaP (diphtheria, tetanus, and acellular pertussis). Allergic reactions to the MMR vaccine are most likely to be caused by an allergy to the gelatin in the vaccine rather than to any other component in the vaccine. As a general rule, any person who has experienced an allergic reaction after eating gelatin food products (e.g., Jell-O) should not be given any of the above vaccines. However, as is the case with egg-containing vaccines in egg-allergic people, it may be possible to give gelatin-containing vaccines to gelatin-allergic people under the direct supervision of a physician.

60. I had facial flushing, nausea, and diarrhea after eating tuna. Is this an allergy to fish?

This reaction could certainly represent an allergic reaction to tuna. Fish allergy, as noted in Question 53, is one of the more common foods to which adults become allergic. Certainly, if you have experienced systemic reactions, including hives, flushing, gastrointestinal symptoms, wheezing, throat swelling, or dizziness after eating some type of fish, you should undergo blood or skin allergy testing to a panel of different types of fish to determine whether you are allergic to these foods. In the event that these tests are negative, there is an alternative explanation for these symptoms. Occasionally, when tuna, mackerel, mahi-mahi, or bluefish become contaminated with certain bacteria (usually *Proteus* or *Klebsiella*), histamine is formed in the meat of the fish in large quantities. Eating the spoiled fish produces a sharp peppery taste and a burning feeling in the inside of the mouth, followed by nausea, vomiting, facial flushing, and headache. This phenomenon, referred to as "scombroid fish poisoning," is self-limited and does not cause a person to become allergic following the episode.

61. Can I be allergic to alcoholic beverages?

Many patients experience acute reactions after drinking beverages containing alcohol. In my own experience, the most frequently described adverse effects of alcohol can be attributed to alcohol intolerance, with exaggeration of the expected physical effects. The symptoms of alcohol intolerance may include headache, rapid heartbeat, nausea, vomiting, heartburn, abdominal pain, nasal congestion, and flushing. These last two symptoms, nasal congestion and flushing, are almost universally due to the vasodilating effects of alcohol in the

The symptoms of alcohol intolerance may include headache, rapid heartbeat, nausea, vomiting, heartburn, abdominal pain, nasal congestion, and flushing.

nasal mucous membrane and skin. A higher-than-expected percentage of people of Asian descent appear to be more susceptible to this flushing effect, and it is believed to be caused by an inability to metabolize alcohol completely. As this syndrome does not represent an IgE-mediated allergic reaction, there is no diagnostic test, such as a skin or blood test, that can be performed for confirming this disorder.

Occasionally, people will experience systemic reactions with hives, wheezing, and/or throat swelling. In these cases, the most likely explanation would be intolerance of sulfites, which are usually found in white wine. Less commonly, allergy to other ingredients, such as grapes in wine, grains in beers (such as hops, barley, rye, corn, or wheat), and yeast, may be present. In cases of possible allergy to a component in the alcoholic beverage, an allergy skin or blood test can be performed. A last possible explanation for some of these symptoms, particularly flushing and headache, is histamine in red wine. While there is a variable amount of histamine in red wine, it is debatable whether this chemical is the cause of these symptoms. Irrespective of which type of alcohol is consumed or which mechanism is at play, the only reliable solution to all of these problems is to avoid alcohol.

62. Is there any relationship between seasonal hay fever and food allergies?

Certain raw fruits and vegetables may cause patients to develop itching of the lips, mouth, and throat. This syndrome, called **oral allergy syndrome**, is caused by specific proteins in the foods (including melons, bananas, and apples). Importantly, these proteins are heat-sensitive and can be rendered nonallergenic by cooking the food. For example, patients who have oral allergy syndrome after eating a raw apple will be able to

Oral allergy syndrome

A food allergy to certain raw fruits and vegetables that causes itching and occasionally swelling of the oral cavity.

Table 8   Examples of Foods and Pollens That Share Proteins

Pollen	Food
Ragweed	Melons, bananas
Birch tree	Apple, pear, hazelnut, carrot, potato, celery, kiwi
Grass	Peaches, celery
Mugwort	Celery

tolerate baked apple pie without symptoms. Due to proteins that are present in both these raw foods as well as certain seasonal pollens, patients who have seasonal hay fever caused by the pollen will develop symptoms after eating the food. Examples of this allergenic cross-reactivity are shown in **Table 8**.

63. Can food allergies cause heartburn?

Heartburn is caused by gastric acid rising up out of the stomach and into the esophagus, causing irritation and inflammation. This condition, referred to medically as **gastroesophageal reflux disease (GERD)**, usually occurs because of loosening of the sphincter muscle where the esophagus enters the stomach and may be present in people of all ages. A number of foods and beverages may cause or aggravate GERD, including caffeine-containing drinks (especially coffee), alcohol, and greasy and spicy foods. All of these foods are thought to provoke acid reflux by causing the esophageal sphincter to become more relaxed than usual, allowing stomach contents to enter the esophagus. It must be emphasized that the effects of these foods are not due to allergy.

However, there is another esophageal condition in which allergic inflammation occurs in the esophagus, referred to as **eosinophilic esophagitis**. This diagnosis is usually suspected when a patient does not improve with appropriate treatment for acid reflux, such as antacids,

Gastroesophageal reflux disease (GERD)

A condition in which gastric acid rises from the stomach into the esophagus, causing irritation and inflammation.

Eosinophilic esophagitis

Allergic inflammation that occurs in the esophagus, occasionally as a result of food allergy.

H$_2$ blocking drugs (e.g., ranitidine), or proton-pump inhibitors (e.g., omeprazole). Because these patients do not usually respond to appropriate reflux therapy, it is important for a gastroenterologist to confirm the diagnosis of eosinophilic esophagitis by visual endoscopic inspection and biopsy of the esophagus. In this disease, food allergens may play an important role in causing inflammation. Accurate determination of which foods are acting as allergens requires a combination of prick/puncture skin tests followed by delayed-type hypersensitivity testing (patch testing). Patch testing involves the placement of a sample of pulverized food into a small metal holder which is then taped onto the patient's skin for 2 days. At the end of the 2-day period, the container of food is removed and the area of skin in contact with the food is inspected for redness and/or blistering. In patients in whom a food is identified as a relevant trigger, avoidance of the implicated food(s) may have a profound effect upon the esophageal inflammation and symptoms of reflux.

James's comment:

I started having bad heartburn last year, and it seemed to get worse after eating. Occasionally, during a spell of heartburn, I would feel a squeezing pain in my chest that got a little better with Tums. My doctor told me to stop having coffee and other caffeinated drinks and to eat no later than 7 PM. He started me on Zantac twice a day, which didn't really help. After a couple of weeks, he switched the medicine to Prilosec twice a day, but I was still having heartburn and pain. I was referred to a gastroenterologist, who did an endoscopy and took a biopsy that showed something called "eosinophilic esophagitis." She referred me to an allergist, who first did a skin prick test, which was negative to every food. The allergist then did a special test called a "food patch test," which was left on my back for 2 days and showed that

I had an allergy to soy and milk. Since stopping those two foods, which I used to eat all of the time, my heartburn has gradually gone away.

64. What is the best test for diagnosing food allergies?

The most important component in diagnosing allergy to a food is the patient's history. A food allergy is most often suspected when a particular item was eaten prior to the onset of acute symptoms. In some cases, the implicated food was eaten by itself, making it easy to identify the probable source of symptoms. In many cases, however, several foods were eaten as part of the same meal, making it more difficult to sort out which food the patient reacted to. When food-induced symptoms occur frequently without an obvious consistent trigger, a daily diary may be very helpful. The patient records the timing of meals, amount of food eaten, how the food was prepared, all activities (such as exercise) that were performed in relationship to the reaction, and the symptoms and duration of the reaction.

Following the initial history and possibly the extended use of a diary, allergy testing should be performed to confirm which food caused the reaction. Generally, testing can be limited to those foods that were eaten 2 or fewer hours prior to the onset of symptoms. In cases of mild food reactions, allergists perform prick/puncture skin testing. If the prick/puncture test is negative to a food, the person is considered to have no allergy to that food. Intradermal skin testing to foods should never be performed, either as an initial test or as a secondary test in patients who have negative prick/puncture tests. When used as an initial test, the large amount of allergen injected with this type of test can induce a dangerous systemic reaction. When used as a secondary test,

The most important component in diagnosing allergy to a food is the patient's history.

intradermal tests yield very nonspecific results such that a positive result is just as likely to occur in a patient who has no allergy as it is in a patient who has a proven allergy. In patients with histories of more severe reactions to foods, the physician may advise that you undergo blood allergy testing for safety reasons. The most reliable blood test for diagnosing food allergies is the ImmunoCap assay which determines the amount of IgE directed at specific foods. Although this blood test for food allergies is not quite as sensitive as prick/puncture skin testing, it is still an extremely accurate test, which yields valid results. Tests that determine the presence of IgG to foods have not proven useful in diagnosing food allergy.

65. If I am allergic to peanuts, how careful do I have to be?

Peanuts are commonly used as an ingredient in a large variety of processed foods, particularly baked goods, ice cream, and candies. As even trace amounts of peanuts may provoke an allergic reaction in a peanut-allergic person, these foods should be strictly avoided. Frequently, food manufacturing equipment used to process sunflower seeds and tree nut butters are used to process peanut-containing foods, thus resulting in possible contamination of these foods with peanut protein. In the event that a peanut-allergic patient does consume a small amount of peanut protein, the possibility of a reaction will be most closely related to the amount of peanut eaten, the patient's level of allergic sensitivity, and the type of organ system involvement that has occurred in the past (e.g., mild hives versus severe anaphylaxis). If a patient is aware of having eaten a noticeable amount of peanuts, is highly peanut-sensitive, and has a history of major systemic symptoms after consuming peanuts, epinephrine should be administered by injection and the patient should be closely observed over the next few hours. If symptoms do develop despite the administration of epinephrine, the patient should be given another dose of epinephrine within 15 minutes of the first dose and should then be taken to the nearest emergency room. If symptoms appear to be progressing, particularly if there is involvement of breathing or severe dizziness, the patient should be transported by ambulance.

Epinephrine

A naturally occurring hormone that is administered as an injectable drug that is used to stop anaphylactic allergic reactions.

66. I am highly allergic to peanuts, and a recent allergy test also showed small reactions to soy and wheat, even though I can eat these foods without developing symptoms. Do I need to avoid soy and wheat?

This scenario brings up a couple of very important points regarding food allergy. First, the peanut is a member of the legume family, which also includes peas, soybeans, and other types of beans. If a patient is allergic to one member of the legume family (e.g., peanuts), there is a high probability that he or she will have a positive skin or blood allergy test to another legume. However, the positive test does not indicate that the patient will have clinical symptoms when that other food is eaten. It is therefore not surprising that despite a positive skin test to soy, a patient may be able to eat this food without any difficulty. Wheat, on the other hand, is not at all related to the legume family. However, when a large panel of food allergy tests (skin or blood) is performed, it is not unusual to see occasional small positive reactions to foods that are eaten without developing symptoms. For this reason, it is best not to undergo large numbers of allergy tests to foods that the person has been able to tolerate without problems.

67. If I'm allergic to shrimp, can I eat other shellfish?

The protein most often linked to shellfish allergy, called "tropomyosin," is found in all types of shellfish, including abalone, clams, cockle, crab, crayfish, lobster, mollusks, mussels, octopus, oysters, scallops, shrimp, snails, and squid. The likelihood that a person who is allergic to one type of shellfish, such as shrimp, is allergic to another, such as lobster, is approximately 75%. Although people of any age can develop a shellfish allergy, it occurs most commonly in adults. Shellfish allergy is also more common in women. After taking a careful history, allergy testing to shellfish by skin testing or blood testing is the most reliable way to tell if the person is truly allergic. Adverse reactions to shellfish are also sometimes caused by a nonallergic reaction, such as food poisoning.

The likelihood that a person who is allergic to one type of shellfish, such as shrimp, is allergic to another, such as lobster, is approximately 75%.

68. Do food allergies go away, and, if not, are they curable with treatment?

Fortunately, many of the food allergies that occur in infancy and early childhood resolve spontaneously between the ages of 3 and 5 years. Prominent examples of these foods include milk, soy, and eggs. However, peanut allergy, which usually also occurs in early life, has a very low chance of going away as the patient grows older. Food allergies that develop later in life, such as fish and shellfish, also have a very low rate of spontaneous resolution. Currently, no treatment exists to cure persistent food allergies. A number of specialized clinical centers are actively at work to develop oral challenge protocols that will help induce food tolerance. Until this becomes an established clinical procedure, we do not recommend that patients undergo any form of food desensitization, whether it be by injection, pill, or liquid that is either swallowed or instilled under the tongue.

69. Do I need to avoid shellfish if I am sensitive to radiocontrast media?

Injectable dye, also referred to as **radiocontrast media (RCM)**, is used in a wide variety of x-ray studies, including angiograms, computed tomography (CT) scans, and intravenous pyelograms. Reactions to RCM have been reported to occur in up to 13% of patients receiving intravenous contrast. More often than not, the reactions are mild and consist of flushing, dizziness, and nausea. Less than 2% of people receiving contrast will have more severe reactions, which may include diffuse hives, vomiting, and occasionally throat swelling or a drop in blood pressure. People who are at higher risk for reactions to RCM include women, the elderly, those with past reactions to RCM, patients with histories of asthma, allergies, and heart disease, and people taking beta-blocker drugs.

> **Radiocontrast medium (RCM)**
> Dye injected into a person to improve visibility of internal structures during an x-ray procedure (e.g., intravenous pyelogram for detection of kidney stones).

Contrary to popular belief, seafood allergy is in no way connected to RCM reactions. Therefore, if a person has a history of RCM sensitivity, it does not suggest that he or she will be allergic to shrimp or shellfish, or vice versa. The diagnosis of RCM is made strictly based on history, as there is currently no test available that accurately predicts the occurrence of reactions. Prevention of future reactions is the single most important task for the patient and physician. For future procedures involving RCM, the radiologist should use low-ionic, low-osmolarity contrast media in place of high-osmolarity media. In addition, the use of medications, such as prednisone and diphenhydramine, prior to the administration of RCM may help greatly in reducing the incidence and severity of reactions.

70. Does food allergy cause autism?

Autism is a disorder that affects brain development in children and causes problems with social interaction and communication skills. In recent years, investigators

> **Autism**
> A neural developmental disorder characterized by impaired social and communication skills.

have sought to understand the role of food allergies in causing or worsening the severity of autism. Specifically, gluten (a wheat protein) and casein (a milk protein) have been occasionally blamed for worsening symptoms in some children by contributing to immune dysfunction. Many other foods are blamed for worsening autism as well, including eggs, tomatoes, eggplant, avocado, red peppers, soy, and corn. Based on these precepts, autistic children may be placed on severely restricted diets for prolonged periods of time.

Clinical studies reveal that allergy skin and blood tests, which assess the presence of IgE antibodies to these foods are usually negative, and most of these children do not experience typical symptoms of food allergies. In addition, studies of gluten- and casein-free diets in autistic children have not met with strict scientific scrutiny and have yielded questionable information. Recently, a Cochrane analysis on this subject found only one small, well-designed study that showed some improvement in autistic traits in the children receiving a gluten- and casein-free diet. Studies of larger numbers of children are needed to confirm the results of this small study. It should be kept in mind that severely limiting a child's dietary intake may lead to nutritional deficiencies. Be sure to contact your child's physicians before starting a strict diet in a young child.

71. What is celiac disease?

Celiac disease

A digestive condition that results from eating gluten, characterized by diarrhea, pain, and intestinal malabsorption.

Celiac disease is a digestive condition caused by eating gluten, which is a protein found in bread, pasta, cookies, pizza crust, and many other foods containing wheat, barley, or rye. If you have celiac disease and eat foods containing gluten, an immune reaction occurs in your small intestine, causing damage to the surface of your small intestine and an inability to absorb certain nutrients.

Eventually, the decreased absorption of nutrients may lead to vitamin deficiencies that cause damage to the brain, peripheral nervous system, bones, liver, and other organs.

If someone in your immediate family has celiac disease, chances are 5–15% that you may have it as well. The disease often manifests after some form of trauma such as an infection, a physical injury, pregnancy, severe psychologic stress, or surgery. The most common symptoms consist of intermittent diarrhea, abdominal pain, and bloating. Other diseases that may also present with these symptoms include irritable bowel syndrome, gastric ulcers, Crohn's disease, and parasitic infections of the intestines.

Occasionally, people with celiac disease may have no gastrointestinal symptoms at all, and may present in less obvious ways, including anemia, skin rash, weight loss, general weakness, stunted growth (in children), and osteoporosis. People with celiac disease carry higher than normal levels of certain antibodies, including anti-gliadin, anti-endomysium, and anti-tissue transglutaminase. Blood tests are routinely available, which can detect the levels of these antibodies and can be used to initially detect people who are most likely to have celiac disease and who may need further testing. To confirm the diagnosis, your doctor may need to microscopically examine a small portion of intestinal tissue to check for damage to the intestinal lining. This procedure is called a biopsy. To do this, your doctor inserts a thin, flexible tube (endoscope) through your mouth, esophagus, and stomach into your small intestine and takes a sample of intestinal tissue.

A trial of a gluten-free diet can also confirm a diagnosis, but it is important that you not start such a diet before seeking a medical evaluation. Doing so may change the results of blood tests and biopsies so that they appear to be normal.

72. How is celiac disease treated?

No treatment can cure celiac disease. However, you can effectively manage celiac disease through changing your diet. Once gluten is removed from your diet, inflammation in your small intestine will begin to resolve, usually within a few weeks. Even a small amount of gluten is enough to cause symptoms and complications, which means all foods or food ingredients made from many grains must be avoided.

Because a gluten-free diet needs to be strictly followed, you may wish to consult a registered dietitian who is experienced in instructing patients regarding gluten-free diets (see **Table 9**). Foods that contain gluten include any type of wheat (including farina, graham flour, semolina, and durum), barley, rye, bulgur, Kamut, kasha, matzo meal, spelt, and triticale. Amaranth, buckwheat, and quinoa are gluten-free as grown, but they may be contaminated

Table 9   Which Grains and Starches Contain Gluten?

Gluten-Containing	Gluten-Free
Wheat	Amaranth
Farina	Buckwheat
Graham flour	Quinoa
Semolina	Oats
Durum	Rice
Barley	Soy
Rye	Corn
Bulgur	Potato
Kamut	
Kasha	
Matzo meal	
Spelt	
Triticale	

by other grains during harvesting and processing, so be sure that the label says gluten-free or manufactured in a gluten-free facility. **Cross-contamination** may also occur if gluten-free products are prepared in unwashed bowls previously containing gluten products. Oats may not be harmful for most people with celiac disease, but oat products are frequently contaminated with wheat, so it is best to avoid oats as well. Most commercially available baked goods contain gluten and should be strictly avoided unless they are labeled as gluten-free. Flours that are usually safest include rice, soy, corn, and potato. If your nutritional deficiencies are severe, you may need to take vitamin and mineral supplements.

Once a gluten-free diet is started, complete healing of the intestine may take several months in younger people and 2–3 years in older people. Most people with celiac disease who follow a gluten-free diet have a complete recovery. Rarely, people with severely damaged small intestines do improve with a gluten-free diet. When diet is not effective, treatment often includes medications to help control intestinal inflammation and other conditions resulting from malabsorption.

73. Is there any way to prevent children from becoming food allergic?

Over the past 10 to 15 years, researchers have sought ways to prevent the development of food allergy in children. A large number of interventions have been tried in parents who are at increased risk for having allergic children, including dietary restriction in the mother (during pregnancy and breast-feeding), strict adherence to a breast milk diet for the infant, and dietary restriction in the infant after food is introduced. While some of the studies have shown that food allergy was initially reduced in the newborn, by 2 years of age the prevalence

Cross-contamination

Transfer of a harmful food element from one food product to another, often occurring inadvertently during food production or preparation.

was comparable to children who did not undergo the dietary interventions. Currently, researchers are looking at new ways to reduce food allergy in high-risk babies. Preliminary findings suggest that early introduction of peanuts into the newborn's diet may actually block the development of a peanut allergy. While this is a very exciting and important prospect, it cannot be recommended until large, rigorous trials confirm these observations.

74. If I am allergic to peanuts, should I avoid all nuts?

Almost half of people who are allergic to peanuts are also allergic to tree nuts, such as almonds, Brazil nuts, walnuts, hazelnuts, macadamias, pistachios, pecans, and cashews. People who are allergic to one tree nut are often allergic to at least one other tree nut. Tree nut reactions can be severe, even with small exposures, and research has shown that peanuts and tree nuts are the two leading causes of fatal food allergy reactions. Given these considerations, I recommend to patients that any tree nut that is skin-test positive be removed from the diet.

75. What can we do at home to prevent serious allergic reactions to foods, and how do I treat it if it happens?

Several important steps can protect a patient with serious food allergies from having future reactions. These steps include:

1. Remove all sources of food that the patient is allergic to. Even trace amounts of a food protein can cause a severe reaction in some people. It can be particularly challenging to avoid foods that frequently show up in food items as hidden ingredients, such as peanuts. Therefore, always read food labels carefully before

purchasing a food item. Companies are required to clearly label any product that contains even small amounts of a food product. Periodic alerts published by the Food Allergy and Anaphylaxis Network are very helpful in updating patients regarding hidden sources of food allergens.

2. Be careful when dining out. Most inadvertent exposures to allergenic foods occur while eating in restaurants or in friends' homes. When you eat at restaurants, always check to make sure that food ordered by the allergic patient was not cooked in the same pans, oils, or utensils used to prepare foods that are allergenic to that patient (i.e., cross-contamination). Tell everyone who handles the food that the allergic person eats, including waiters in restaurants and cafeteria workers at school, about the food allergy. If the manager or owner of a restaurant cannot accommodate your request for allergen-free food preparation, you probably should not eat there.

3. Do not eat foods with an unknown list of ingredients. For children with food allergies, it is very important to make all lunches and snacks that are taken to school or any outing away from home.

4. For children, talk to the day care supervisor or school principal, and work with the school and family friends to create a food allergy emergency action plan.

5. Wear a Medic-Alert bracelet to identify yourself as having a life-threatening allergy to food.

6. Epinephrine is the single most important treatment for food-induced anaphylaxis. People with histories of systemic reactions to foods should have epinephrine available at all times, including in their backpack or purse, home, school nursing office, and car(s).

Epinephrine is the single most important treatment for food-induced anaphylaxis. People with histories of systemic reactions to foods should have epinephrine available at all times, including in their backpack or purse, home, school nursing office, and car(s).

A very convenient method for injecting epinephrine is the EpiPen Autoinjector™. By pressing the pre-loaded injection device firmly against the thigh, a measured amount of epinephrine is injected through fabric and into the muscle. It is available as an EpiPen Jr™ (0.15 ml for children weighing 33 to 66 pounds) and EpiPen (0.30 ml for patients weighing more than 66 pounds). Other commercially available devices for injecting epinephrine include the AnaPen™, Ana-Kit™, and Twinject™. Epinephrine should be administered immediately when a person first begins to experience a systemic allergic reaction to a food. In addition, if a person realizes that they have just ingested a food that they are highly allergic to, they should administer the epinephrine prophylactically to avert a major reaction. Oral antihistamines are not an effective means of treating or preventing a systemic allergic reaction to foods.

PART FOUR

Insect Sting Allergy

Which insects can cause insect sting allergy,
and what are the symptoms?

If I have a history of severe bee sting allergy,
what should I do the next time I am stung?

Do allergy shots work for insect allergy?

More . . .

76. Which insects can cause insect sting allergy, and what are the symptoms?

Several insects belonging to order Hymenoptera are capable of injecting venom into humans and animals by stinging or biting. These insects include honeybees, bumblebees, hornets, wasps, yellow jackets, and fire ants, all of which are currently found in the United States as well as in most other land areas of the globe. Their venom, which they use to kill or paralyze other insects, is composed of proteins and other substances that are capable of causing allergic reactions. After a sting or bite by any of these insects, a normal response consists of a small, localized area of redness and itching. Some patients develop large local skin reactions that may be several inches in diameter and last for several days. These local responses represent a mild form of allergy to insect stings; rarely do these patients develop systemic reactions following future stings. Patients with a greater degree of allergy to insect stings present with systemic symptoms, including hives, throat swelling, wheezing, dizziness, abdominal pain, nausea and vomiting, diarrhea, and/or a drop in blood pressure.

77. How do I know what type of insect stung me?

It is often very difficult to determine the source of a sting. This is why it is recommended that patients who have experienced an allergic reaction to an insect sting undergo testing to a complete panel of stinging insects. Despite this difficulty, there are some clues that will help a victim of a sting determine the type of insect that was involved.

Honeybees are usually nonaggressive and only sting when their hive is threatened, or if they are struck or stepped on. Most bee stings occur in people who are barefoot while outdoors. Africanized honeybees (killer bees) are much more aggressive than domestic honeybees and frequently attack people in swarms who approach their hive. Due to their ability to dominate other bees, Africanized bees have become increasingly common throughout the United States. Because their stingers are barbed, all honeybees will leave their stinger in the skin of their victim, limiting the honeybee to one sting. As the stinger is pulled out of the bee's body, the bee loses some of its internal organs and dies in the process. Bumblebees are very large and scary to encounter, but they are not usually aggressive and rarely sting unless provoked. As they fly slowly and buzz loudly, they are easy to identify from a distance. Bumblebee stingers have no barbs and remain with the bee after stinging, allowing the bee to sting multiple times.

Wasps live in honeycomb-like nests often under the overhangs of houses. Wasps tend to be nonaggressive, although they sting when disturbed. They do not leave a stinger in their victims, so they are able to sting repeatedly. Yellow jackets live in nests on the ground and are the most aggressive of all of the stinging insects. Like wasps, they are able to sting multiple times. They live by scavenging for food and are commonly found around trash cans, dumpsters, and picnics, and are prone to seek out cans and bottles of sweet beverages. This tendency to climb into beverage containers may result in stings on the lips, inside the mouth, or on the tongue. Yellow-faced and white-faced hornets live in trees and shrubs in "paper-mâché" nests. They will attack their victims when provoked and are also able to sting multiple times.

78. I was stung by a bee recently. Do I need to be allergy tested?

The first step in establishing whether a patient is allergic to insect stings is a detailed history. Once the type of insect and severity of the reaction have been characterized, allergy skin testing may be performed to confirm whether or not the patient is allergic to any of the stinging insects. All people, regardless of any age, should undergo testing if they have symptoms of a systemic reaction after a sting. This group stands to benefit most from accurate diagnosis and treatment, as 60–70% of patients with a history of a systemic reaction are at risk for similar future reactions after stings. While the chance of a reaction with a future sting does decrease over time, it still remains at about 20% many years after the last sting. Allergy testing to insect venom is not needed if a person was stung in the past but never had any allergic symptoms, if a child under 16 years of age has had only skin symptoms such as hives and/or swelling after a sting, or if a child or adult has had only a large local reaction. However, in some cases a physician may elect to test these patients, particularly if they are at high risk for future stings. In addition, people should not be tested if they have never been stung or if there is only a family history of a reaction to a sting.

79. If I have a history of severe bee sting allergy, what should I do the next time I am stung?

If bees are flying around you after the sting, always stay calm and avoid swatting at them; this will encourage additional stings. After the sting, you should quickly leave the area. When a bee stings, it releases a chemical that attracts other bees that may then sting. Once you are in a clear area, you should attempt to remove the stinger. This can only be done when the insect is a honey bee, since honeybees are the only Hymenoptera that leave their stingers behind. The stinger is best removed with some stiff material, such as a piece of cardboard or a credit card. After removal, epinephrine should be given immediately, without waiting to see whether symptoms develop (see Question 75). After the epinephrine has been given, you should go immediately to the closest emergency room to be observed and treated.

80. How can I keep from getting stung in the future?

For an allergic patient, there are a number of ways to prevent future insect stings. Suggestions include:

- Avoid using perfumes, scented soaps, and other sweet or pungent body products.
- Avoid wearing bright colors that might attract bees.
- Stay away from blooming flowers when you are outdoors.
- Avoid eating sweet foods while your are outdoors.
- Consider wearing protective clothing when outdoors, including long-sleeved shirts, gloves, and hats.
- Wear shoes when walking outside.
- When driving, keep your windows rolled up.
- Have a professional inspection performed, and remove bee hives or other sources of stinging insects near your home.
- Always be prepared for the possibility of a future sting by carrying emergency epinephrine with you.
- Purchase a medical identification bracelet (Medic-Alert) that identifies you as having an insect sting allergy. This identification is extremely important in the event that you have a serious reaction and cannot communicate.
- Discuss with your doctor the possibility of starting allergy shot therapy to reduce your hypersensitivity to stinging insects.

81. Do allergy shots work for insect allergy?

Allergy shots for insect stings, also called venom immunother-apy, are the most effective known treatment to prevent allergic reactions to stings from honeybees, yellow jackets, hornets, paper wasps, and fire ants.

Immunotherapy

A form of treatment for allergic diseases in which the patient receives increasing amounts of the substance that they are allergic to, resulting in tolerance.

Allergy shots for insect stings, also called venom **immunotherapy**, are the most effective known treatment to prevent allergic reactions to stings from honeybees, yellow jackets, hornets, paper wasps, and fire ants. Venom immunotherapy is offered to all patients who have had anaphylaxis following a sting and to adults who have had acute hives after a sting. In addition, patients with very large, aggressive local reactions who have positive skin tests may be considered as candidates, as shots have been recently shown to reduce the intensity of these reactions and a sting to the neck or face could have dire consequences. If a person has no symptoms of allergic reactions to insect stings but is tested and found positive to a venom skin test, the chance of developing anaphylaxis with future stings is approximately 17%. In this circumstance, because a positive test now exists, venom allergy shots should be offered, given the small but significant chance of a severe allergic reaction in the future.

The therapy is started using extremely small amounts of venom from all of the insects that the patient is allergic to. Levels of these venoms are increased over time. After 4–6 months of weekly injections, most patients reach the highest tolerated dose of venom, which is referred to by allergists as the maintenance dose. Patients will usually receive the maintenance dose every 4 weeks for approximately 1 year, then every 6–8 weeks for 3–5 more years. Patients who are at high risk for future stings (e.g., forest rangers, landscape designers) may benefit from receiving their initial immunotherapy more quickly, thus acquiring protection against future stings. This treatment program, which is called "rush immunotherapy," consists of administering several shots each day, 2–3 days per week over a few weeks.

Venom shots should always be given in a doctor's office. It is normal to remain in the doctor's office for at least 30 minutes after receiving an allergy injection in order to observe for any possible systemic reactions.

Immunotherapy for insect stings significantly reduces your chances of having another severe systemic allergic reaction from 60% to less than 3%. It is not clear exactly how effective the protection against future stings is after the treatment has ended. In about 80–90% of cases, patients will still be protected against systemic reactions even if allergy tests show some remaining allergy to the venom. Venom immunotherapy is safe if the shots are given correctly and the most common side effect is redness and warmth at the injection site. Some people may experience large, local reactions that include itching, hives, or swelling of the skin. Less commonly, a shot may lead to systemic symptoms such as hives, itching, or difficulty breathing. For this reason, venom immunotherapy should always be administered by a physician familiar with this type of therapy and who is prepared to treat a systemic reaction.

PART FIVE

Drug Allergy

What is a drug allergy, and what are the most
common symptoms?

If I am allergic to penicillin, will I be allergic
to other antibiotics?

Will a skin test tell me if I am allergic
to a medication?

More...

82. What is a drug allergy, and what are the most common symptoms?

Adverse effects from drugs are extremely common and can be divided into two broad categories. **Drug intolerance** represents a pharmacologic effect of a medication that creates undesirable symptoms. A good example is nausea and vomiting after taking codeine cough syrup or insomnia after using pseudoephedrine. These intolerances do not represent allergies and will be relatively consistent each time the drug is taken. The other major category of reactions is an **immunologic sensitivity** induced by the drug, broadly referred to as a drug allergy. Drug allergies are much less common, accounting for about 5–10% of adverse reactions to medications.

In order for patients to develop an allergy to a drug, they need to have taken the medication before. Once they have taken the drug on one or more occasions, their immune system is then able to form a specific type of response to the drug that causes them to have allergic symptoms when they take it again. The most common mechanism by which the immune system reacts to a drug is the development of IgE antibodies. These antibodies lead to allergic reactions which come on very quickly, usually within minutes to hours after taking a drug. The severity of a reaction is related to the amount of drug taken, the route of delivery (injectable medications cause worse reactions than oral), and the level of allergic sensitivity. The most common symptoms caused by an IgE reaction to a drug are itching of the skin along with hives and/or swelling. Occasionally, patients will develop severe generalized reactions that extend to other organs beside the skin, consisting of wheezing, throat swelling, abdominal cramping, diarrhea, dizziness, and possibly a large drop in blood pressure (shock).

Drug intolerance

Adverse side effects of a drug that are not mediated by the immune system.

Immunologic sensitivity

Sensitivity to a substance which is caused by components of the immune system, including antibodies and lymphocytes.

Other immunologic reactions to drugs are not related to IgE antibodies but are instead caused by immune cells. These reactions, referred to as cell-mediated immune reactions, typically consist of a diffuse pinpoint rash that involves much of the body and begins several days after starting the medication. Another less common mechanism is caused by IgE antibodies, called an "immune complex reaction." The immune complexes, which consist of a clump of IgE antibodies bound to the drug, circulate in the bloodstream and then become lodged in body tissues, particularly the skin and kidney. The small hemorrhages caused by these immune complexes are manifested as small bloody dots or bruises in the skin or bleeding into the kidney.

83. I received a Novacaine shot from my dentist and felt very dizzy and sick to my stomach. Am I allergic to Novacaine?

True allergic reactions to local anesthetics such as lidocaine (Novacaine) are extremely rare; in fact, some experts doubt that these substances are capable of causing true allergic reactions. Most often, patients will experience what is called a "vasovagal reaction," which is a type of response that often occurs following any type of injection or blood draw. In a vasovagal reaction, the person may have paleness of the skin, sweating, dizziness, and nausea, often followed by fainting. The physician may suspect this type of reaction because there is a characteristic slowing of the pulse, whereas in a true allergic reaction the pulse usually speeds up. This type of reaction is easily treated by lying the patient down and lifting the feet. If the local anesthetic is injected with epinephrine, which is typically added to the anesthetic to slow the absorption of the drug into the bloodstream, patients may feel "racy" and have a rapid heart rate or skipped heartbeats. Rarely, a patient may be hypersensitive to a preservative, such as sulfites, which are present in the injectable. An allergist may provide useful information in these cases and can perform allergy skin testing, if indicated, to help better define the cause of the reaction.

84. If I am allergic to penicillin, will I be allergic to other antibiotics?

Penicillin and its derivatives (e.g., amoxicillin, methicillin, and dicloxacillin) are the most commonly encountered antibiotics resulting in allergic reactions. These drugs contain a structure referred to as the beta-lactam ring, which is also present in other classes of antibiotics, including cephalosporins (e.g., cephalexin, cefuroxime), carbapenems (imipenem and meropenem, which are both intravenous drugs), and monobactams (aztreonam, which is also an intravenous drug). Because all of these groups of antibiotics share a common chemical structure, there is concern that reacting to one drug will predispose a person to a reaction to a related drug (called "immunologic cross-reactivity"). Certainly, when patients are allergic to an antibiotic in a specific group, (e.g., Penicillin VK, which is oral penicillin), there is a very high chance that they will react to another medication in that group (e.g., dicloxacillin, which is a penicillin derivative). When individuals who are truly allergic to a penicillin derivative (see Question 87) take one of the cephalosporin drugs, very few of them will have an allergic reaction. However, in order to be as safe as possible, we recommend that cephalosporins be avoided in patients who are truly penicillin-allergic unless no other good antibiotic option is available. While carbapenem drugs should be similarly avoided in patients who are penicillin-allergic, aztreonam can be safely given to patients who have a penicillin allergy. There is no other known allergy link between penicillin and other classes of antibiotics, such as sulfa (e.g., Bactrim), quinolones (e.g., Levaquin), and macrolides (e.g., erythromycin, Biaxin).

85. Will a skin test tell me if I am allergic to a medication?

Currently, there are very few valid skin tests for the diagnosis of drug allergy. Drugs for which there are accepted testing protocols include penicillin and Amoxicillin, local anesthetics, muscle relaxants for anesthesia (suxamethonium), and insulin. While other drugs may be tested, there is less experience with these agents and the results may be more difficult to interpret. Penicillin skin testing, which is the most frequently performed antibiotic skin test, typically consists of a battery of tests to penicillin, amoxicillin, and the metabolic breakdown products of penicillin. If these tests are all negative, the risk of having an immediate allergic reaction to penicillin, such as hives or anaphylaxis, is on the order of only 3% or less.

86. If I am allergic to aspirin, is there any way I can take it?

Aspirin, which is a type of medication known as non-steroidal anti-inflammatory drug (or NSAID), is one of the most commonly used medicines in the world and a very important agent in preventing heart attacks and strokes. Aspirin hypersensitivity usually takes two principal forms: aspirin-exacerbated respiratory disease (AERD) and systemic reactions.

Aspirin
A type of non-steroidal anti-inflammatory drug (NSAID). In addition to pain relief, it is used to prevent heart attacks and strokes.

AERD is the most common type of reaction to aspirin, occurring in patients who suffer from asthma, chronic sinusitis, and nasal polyps. In these patients, even small doses of aspirin or another NSAID will lead to nasal congestion, discharge, and sometimes severe or even life-threatening bronchial constriction with wheezing. In patients with AERD syndrome, a physician can desensitize the patient to aspirin by giving a tiny dose and then increasing it gradually until a full dose is given (usually two tablets, twice daily). This desensitization procedure, which should be done in a hospital setting by specially trained physicians, will not only allow the patient to take aspirin for other purposes (such as prevention of stroke or heart attack), but may also have a beneficial effect on the patient's nasal polyps and asthma.

Systemic reactions to aspirin and NSAIDs present with hives, swelling of the skin, and occasionally throat swelling, or a drop in blood pressure. People who experience hives or more severe systemic reactions as a result of taking NSAIDs are not generally candidates for desensitization.

87. I was told that I had a penicillin allergy as a baby. Should I continue to avoid it as an adult?

As time passes, allergic sensitization to drugs tends to wane, and, in the case of penicillin, 80% of patients are no longer allergic 10 years after having had an initial bona fide allergic reaction.

At least 10% of people in the United States believe they are allergic to penicillin based on reports from their parents that they had reactions as infants. While many of these patients did have rashes while taking some form of penicillin as a baby, particularly amoxicillin, much of the time the rash was due to the virus they were infected with rather than the drug. Therefore, these patients were never truly penicillin-allergic to begin with and were mislabeled from an early age. Some of the patients with rashes after taking a penicillin derivative, particularly those with rapid-onset hives, were truly allergic to penicillin. However, as time passes, allergic sensitization to drugs tends to wane, and, in the case of penicillin, 80% of patients are no longer allergic 10 years after having had an initial bona fide allergic reaction. In most cases, physicians will opt to treat patients with a childhood history of penicillin allergy with alternative antibiotics. However, in some cases, patients believe they have become allergic to multiple types of antibiotics, including penicillin, and do not feel comfortable taking any antibiotic. In these cases, the best thing to do is seek consultation with an allergist for consideration of penicillin skin testing. If the tests are negative, patients should be able to take penicillin or a derivative with a minimal risk of a systemic reaction.

88. After a dental cleaning, I developed swelling of my mouth. I had similar problems while blowing up balloons. What does this indicate?

These two events both involved oral contact with latex rubber. Latex allergy is caused by the development of IgE antibodies to certain proteins found in natural rubber latex, a product manufactured from a milky fluid derived from the rubber tree (*Hevea brasiliensis*) found in Africa and Southeast Asia. Products containing dipped latex such as rubber gloves, balloons, rubber bands, and condoms are a much more common source of allergic symptoms. Hard rubber products, such as athletic shoes, tires, and rubber balls, usually do not cause allergies in most people. In addition, products containing man-made latex, such as latex paint, are unlikely to cause a reaction because they do not contain the naturally occurring latex proteins. Latex allergy may first present as hives or swelling on the skin, or it may lead to systemic symptoms, ranging from sneezing to anaphylaxis.

Some patients have an increased risk for developing latex allergy. The highest risk group is children with spina bifida, which is a birth defect that affects the development of the spine. Children with spina bifida are exposed frequently to latex products during surgical procedures and urinary catheterizations, and about half of them become allergic to latex. The group with the second highest prevalence of latex allergy is healthcare workers, whose primary exposure to latex is in the form of latex gloves. Once allergy to latex is suspected, it can be confirmed either with an allergy skin test, which is performed only by specialists in allergy, or a blood test.

How is latex allergy treated? Latex allergy cannot be cured, so it is critical that latex exposure be reduced. Most latex products have suitable alternatives. If you have a job that involves the use of latex rubber products, talk to your employer and discuss reducing the number of latex products you might come in contact with at work. If you must wear gloves at work, choose gloves made without latex. Vinyl gloves work in many situations, but they are not as effective at protecting you from hepatitis or HIV transmission. Many other types of synthetic gloves work just as well as latex gloves for stopping disease transmission, but they can be more expensive. Stay away from areas of your workplace where other workers may be wearing latex gloves. In addition, request that the people you work with use gloves that are not powdered with cornstarch; the powder becomes easily aerosolized and may result in increased airborne exposure to latex.

In addition to avoiding latex at work, you should inform your healthcare professionals, including your physicians and dentists, about your latex allergy. It is also important to wear a medical alert bracelet. Always keep identification (wallet card or medical bracelet) that clearly alerts others of any allergies you have.

Finally, use nonlatex condoms. If you are allergic to latex, consider using polyurethane or lambskin condoms, or use another type of birth control. However, keep in mind that condoms made of these alternative products do not protect against sexually transmitted diseases as well as latex condoms do. Be sure to read the label on the package to see what the condom is made of and whether it is labeled for disease prevention.

George's comment:

Recently, I was hospitalized for a severe bout of prostatitis, and 20 minutes after inserting a urinary catheter, I started to have itching and swelling of my genital region. At first they thought that the prostate infection was spreading to the skin of my penis, but they later decided that I was having an allergic reaction to the latex in the catheter. After they pulled the catheter out and treated me with medications for the allergy, the redness and itching of my skin improved quickly. A blood test showed that I was allergic to latex, and my team of doctors has decided that I will only receive latex-free catheters in the future.

PART SIX

Allergic Skin Diseases

What causes hives?

What can I do about my child's eczema,
other than medications?

Is it possible to have a skin allergy to sunlight?

More . . .

89. What are hives?

Hives, also called "urticaria," is a type of skin rash that appears as a red, raised welt ranging in size from half an inch to 2 or 3 inches in diameter. Most of the time, hives are intensely itchy but occasionally there can be a burning quality. Typically, an individual hive lesion will last anywhere between an hour up to 12 hours and will resolve without any residual mark or discoloration. When hives last longer than 24 hours, are painful, and leave behind an area of bruising, more serious conditions should be suspected, such as vasculitis (inflammation of the blood vessels).

Hives are caused by the release of histamine and possibly other chemicals, such as leukotrienes, into the superficial skin. These chemicals lead to dilation of blood vessels, which present as swelling in the skin, and stimulation of nerve endings, which causes itching. When this same type of swelling occurs in a deeper level of the skin, the appearance of small, individual hives is lost and the involved area will appear more diffusely swollen. This manifestation is referred to as **angioedema** and most often occurs in parts of the body where the skin is more loosely attached to the underlying connective tissue, such as around the mouth and eyes. Because angioedema occurs at a deeper level of the skin, this type of swelling may take longer to resolve than hives.

90. What causes hives?

Hives and angioedema can be divided into two categories based upon the duration of symptoms: acute and chronic. Acute hives are defined as lesions that come and go for a period of 6 weeks or less, and frequently the outbreak may last for just a few hours or days. Hives that last for a few hours to days are frequently caused by an allergy to a food or an insect sting, while hives that last between several days and a couple of weeks are typically seen with drug allergy or following common viral infections.

Chronic hives and angioedema are defined as lasting for longer than 6 weeks. These patients have hives alone in 40% of cases, hives and angioedema in 40% of cases, and angioedema alone in 20% of cases. In two-thirds of people with chronic hives, no specific cause can be identified (also called "idiopathic"). Approximately 20–30% of patients with chronic hives are considered to have autoimmune hives; these patients have been shown to have antibodies that are directed against molecular targets in their own skin. As a general rule, these patients do not progress to develop other more serious autoimmune diseases, such as systemic lupus erythematosus or rheumatoid arthritis. The next most common cause of chronically recurring hives is a physical stimulus. These triggers include pressure applied to the skin, exposure to cold water or air, or increase in body temperature due to hot water or exercise. The most frequently encountered of these stimuli is physical pressure, also called "dermographia." The underlying basis for these physical causes of hives is not well understood. Other less common causes of chronic hives include systemic diseases such as hormonal disorders (e.g., thyroid disease), and chronic infections (e.g., intestinal parasites). Importantly, when systemic diseases cause hives or angioedema, there are usually other signs and symptoms that suggest the underlying problem in addition to the hives.

In addition to these diseases, there is an extremely rare disorder, called "hereditary angioedema," in which the absence of an important blood protein (C1 esterase inhibitor protein) leads to recurrent acute bouts of deep skin swelling. These patients may have angioedema of the skin, throat, tongue, and/or gastrointestinal tract without any observable hives and the disorder usually becomes symptomatic by the fifth decade of life.

91. Which tests are most important in determining the causes of chronic hives?

The evaluation of chronic hives should always begin with a thorough medical history and physical examination; however, in most cases a cause will not be identified. Most physicians will order a general blood panel, including a complete blood count and white cell differential, erythrocyte sedimentation rate, chemistry panel, thyroid panel, and urinalysis, in order to rule out major systemic diseases. If all of these tests are normal, as they most often are, a number of more specialized tests may be considered.

Autologous serum skin test

Allergy skin test in which a patient's own blood serum is injected into their skin. A positive reaction is most often seen in patients with chronic urticaria and indicates the presence of autoimmune antibodies to certain components in the skin.

First, and most importantly, is a test called the **autologous serum skin test**. As the name implies, blood is taken from the patient and centrifuged to separate the blood cells from the serum; a very small amount of the patient's own serum is then injected intradermally and observed for 15 minutes. If an allergic reaction develops at the site of the injection, it is good evidence that the patient has antibodies in the blood that are attaching to components in the skin and causing the mast cells to release histamine and other chemicals. This procedure is typically done only by an allergist with extensive experience in treating chronic hives. As an alternative to this skin test, a commercial blood test has been developed (Chronic Urticaria Index, IBT Labs), which will detect whether the patient has autoantibodies directed against components in the skin. If the results of either the blood or skin tests are positive, it confirms the diagnosis of autoimmune hives.

If the patient finds that hives or angioedema consistently follow eating, and particularly if the symptoms are more episodic in nature, then allergy skin or blood testing to foods may be useful. In most cases, the foods that are selected for testing are based upon the results of a food diary (see Question 64), in which patients record all episodes of skin lesions along with all foods eaten during a 2- to 4-week period. Those foods that were eaten less than 4 hours before hives would be selected for testing. If patients have daily hives and/or angioedema, however, with no obvious temporal connection to eating, then allergy testing to foods is rarely useful. Patients who have isolated angioedema, particularly those who have had throat or abdominal swelling, should be considered as having possible hereditary angioedema, and special tests of the complement system (C4 complement component and C1 inhibitor functional assay) will need to be performed.

92. What treatments work best for hives?

Initial treatment of acute and chronic hives with or without angioedema relies upon oral H_1 antihistamines. For many years, physicians believed that the older, sedating antihistamines, such as diphenhydramine and hydroxyzine, were more effective for treating hives than the newer nonsedating medications. However, a great body of research has demonstrated that this is not the case. Therefore, I always start the patient on a single daily dose of a nonsedating (loratadine, desloratadine, fexofenadine) or minimally sedating (i.e., cetirizine, levocetirizine) antihistamine. If these are not completely effective in relieving the hives and itching, I will then add an oral H_2 antihistamine, such as ranitidine or cimetidine, in a single daily dose. Most patients recognize these medications as acid blockers for treating stomach ulcers or gastroesophageal reflux disease. However, there are also H_2

histamine receptors in the skin, and blocking these receptors adds significant benefit in controlling the hives. If a combination of H_1 and H_2 antihistamines does not completely control the hives and/or angioedema, the most commonly prescribed third-line medication is montelukast. While montelukast is not currently approved by the Food and Drug Administration (FDA) for the treatment of hives, it has proven helpful in many patients and is generally very well tolerated.

If the combination of these three classes of medications is still not successful and the hives are quite severe, then a course of oral prednisone, 0.5 mg/kg/day is given for 5 to 7 days. In patients with chronic hives, the hives may recur after the prednisone is finished, making it tempting to continue treatment with prednisone. However, prednisone is plagued with many side effects that make it an undesirable choice for long-term use. Alternatives to chronic treatment with prednisone include hydroxycholorquine and cyclosporine, both of which are well tolerated by most patients but require ongoing monitoring to ensure patient safety. Given the possibility of occasionally serious side effects, these medications should only be prescribed by physicians who are experienced in their use and feel that all other alternatives have been considered.

Martin's comment:

I've had hives for the last 4 weeks. Since I didn't have a doctor when they started, I figured it was caused by my soap or detergent or body cream, and I switched those around. I was still having the hives, so I checked for bedbugs or some kind of mite, and everything seemed to be fine with my bedding. A friend told me to take Chlor-Trimeton pills from the pharmacy, and it did help some, but I felt tired all of the time. Since I was now itchy and tired, I saw a doctor at an urgent care, and she recommended over-the-counter pills called loratadine and ranitidine. I took one 10 mg pill of the lorata-dine in the morning and two 75 mg pills of ranitidine twice per day, and after a day I felt 75% better. I'm 25 years old and healthy, and my physical exam was normal, so the doctor told me that she would treat the condition with these pills for a few weeks and see me back before ordering any tests.

93. I've had hives for 6 months, and my doctor has not been able to find out what's causing them. Will they last for the rest of my life?

Fortunately, **chronic idiopathic urticaria** spontaneously resolves over time in the vast majority of patients. After 1 year, 80% of cases will spontaneously resolve; by 2 years, 90% will resolve; and by 5 years, 95% will resolve. These statistics suggest that a small portion of patients will continue to have hives for a very long time, and in my own experience, I have seen a very small number of patients with the disorder for over 15 years without resolution. Often, the severity may change over time, such that the skin lesions become more easily managed as time passes. Following remission, a small but significant group of patients will have relapses after variable periods of time. I have seen patients become hive-free for many years, only to have a recurrence that lasts for months to years. The causes of the recurrence are not well understood, and it is not possible to determine which patients will experience these relapses.

Chronic idiopathic urticaria

Hives that occur for 6 weeks or longer with no known cause.

Chronic idiopathic urticaria spontaneously resolves over time in the vast majority of patients.

94. Are there any medications I should avoid if I have hives or allergic swelling?

It has been estimated that up to one-third of patients with chronic hives and/or angioedema have a sensitivity to aspirin and other nonsteroidal anti-inflammatory drugs (NSAIDs). In these patients, ingestion of these medications leads to acute worsening of their hives and/or angioedema. A small number of these patients will experience more serious systemic reactions following NSAIDs, including throat or tongue swelling. Once the hives have resolved completely for a period of time, the NSAIDs may once again be tolerated without causing hives. Importantly, this sensitivity will occur with all of the NSAIDs, and the more potent the drug, the worse the exacerbation of the hives. Once a patient has this type of reaction to an NSAID, these drugs should be avoided in the future.

Angiotensin converting enzyme (ACE) inhibitor drugs, such as captopril and enalapril, are frequently used to treat hypertension and congestive heart failure as well as to prevent progressive kidney damage in patients with diabetes. It has been advised that individuals with chronic angioedema avoid these drugs as well, since there is a small possibility that these medications may provoke attacks of angioedema.

95. What is allergic eczema?

Allergic eczema, also known as atopic dermatitis, is a chronic itchy skin rash. Atopic dermatitis most often begins in infancy or early childhood and resolves or improves in most cases by age 10 years. In a minority of cases, it can continue into adulthood or may first appear later in life. This rash primarily involves skin on the creases of the arms (where the forearm and upper arm connect), behind the knees, and to a lesser extent on the ankles, wrists, face, neck, and upper chest. In adults, atopic dermatitis can also affect the skin around the eyes, including the eyelids.

The causes of atopic dermatitis are not completely understood, but we do know that persistent allergic inflammation is present in the skin, which contributes to or coexists with a significant defect in the skin's ability to hold on to moisture. Patients with atopic dermatitis are universally sensitive to a number of nonspecific environmental factors, including hot baths or showers, low environmental humidity, soaps and detergents, and prickly fabrics, such as wool.

Along with the above factors, food allergy has a particularly important role in triggering outbreaks of the rash in children, and it has been estimated that up to 25% of children will have an allergic reaction to at least one food. The most common reaction to allergenic foods in patients with atopic dermatitis is redness and itching of the skin, anywhere on the body, and usually occurring within 30 to 60 minutes after eating. The foods that have been implicated in triggering atopic dermatitis most frequently are milk, eggs, wheat, soy, peanuts, and tree nuts. Allergy to these foods is diagnosed as described earlier in this book, by prick/puncture skin testing or blood tests for food IgE. If a number of foods are identified by testing, and it is unclear which are actually triggering the rash, your allergist may recommend oral food challenges. In a food challenge, the food of interest is given to the patient, starting with a very small quantity and gradually increasing the dose. The development of a rash or other symptoms, such as diarrhea, indicates that the patient is allergic to that food. In some cases, avoiding allergenic foods may have a profound effect upon the daily occurrence of rash and itching.

Airborne allergens, such as house dust mites, animal danders, molds, and pollens, have also been shown to aggravate atopic dermatitis. The results are less consistent than those seen with foods. However, in patients with hypersensitivity to avoidable allergens, such as mites, animals, and molds, allergen avoidance measures should be instituted as rigorously as possible in hopes of reducing the need for medications.

Atopic dermatitis frequently runs in families in which other family members have asthma or hay fever. About three out of five infants or children who have atopic dermatitis later develop hay fever and asthma.

96. What can I do about my child's eczema?

In any patient with atopic dermatitis, the first step is to moisturize the skin thoroughly.

In any patient with atopic dermatitis, the first step is to moisturize the skin thoroughly. In the past, physicians routinely recommended avoidance of bathing, believing that it caused further drying of the skin. Most experts now believe that daily bathing is very helpful in restoring moisture to the skin. To help accomplish this, I encourage parents to have their children lie in a tub of tepid water for at least 15 minutes, and if the face is also involved, to place a wet hand towel on the face during that time. I stress the word tepid, as hot water may further irritate dry, itchy skin. While a shower is better than no bathing at all, sitting in a tub is preferable.

After leaving the bath, the skin should be gently patted dry with a soft towel. Immediately after this, a moisturizer should be liberally applied to the entire body, emphasizing areas that are prone to rash. The moisturizer will help seal in the water that has entered the skin during the bath and help prevent future water loss from the skin. The best moisturizer has a high-lipid content, making ointments the best form of moisturizer, followed by creams and then lotions.

Beyond moisturizing, there are other tips patients should consider in treating eczema. In patients living in very dry geographic regions, use of a room humidifier may occasionally be helpful. Irritant avoidance is also very important, which means eliminating heavily perfumed or scented soaps, limiting soap application to the underarms or genital areas or very dirty areas, and completely rinsing all soaps from the body. Equally important is putting all washed clothes through a double rinse cycle in order to remove any residual detergent that might be left in fabric. As noted above (in Question 95), allergenic foods identified by skin or blood tests and possibly oral challenges should be strictly avoided, and environmental control measures aimed at relevant airborne allergens (mites, animals, molds) should be put into place.

When all of the above measures have been taken and the child continues to have a recurring rash, medications will be necessary. In areas of active rash, topical corticosteroids used for 7 to 10 days are very effective in reducing itching, redness, and scaling and expediting the healing of the rash. For the face and neck, it is best to use a low-potency topical steroid (such as hydrocortisone 1% or 2.5% cream) which will usually be effective without causing thinning of the skin. For the body, a medium-potency topical steroid (such as triamcinolone 0.1% ointment) will usually suffice in eliminating signs of inflammation. However, in children with moderate to severe dermatitis, the rash will frequently recur after stopping the steroid. In this situation, use of a nonsteroidal topical anti-inflammatory such as Protopic (tacrolimus ointment) and Elidel (pimecrolimus cream), which may cause the rash to improve markedly for a period of weeks to months before the next recurrence.

Inflammation in atopic dermatitis may be aggravated by bacterial infection of the skin. Children with oozing and crusting of their rash over large amounts of their body may benefit from a 2-week trial of an antibiotic, such as cephalosporin (cephalexin). In situations where the area of infection is very small and localized, a topical antibiotic such as Bactroban (mupirocin) may be adequate.

Occasionally, children are referred to me who have been treated with recurrent courses of oral steroids, such as prednisone, for control of their atopic dermatitis. While these drugs are extremely effective in clearing the rash, I strongly discourage this approach to therapy due to the high occurrence of systemic complications, such as growth impairment, osteoporosis, and cataracts.

97. My child has rough, dry bumps that don't itch on her upper arms and legs. Is this eczema?

Rashes that do not itch are not usually eczema. Rough, dry bumps that feel and look like sandpaper and that occur on the upper arms, legs, and faces of children are commonly due to **keratosis pilaris (KP)**. KP does not usually itch, and it is not usually red or inflamed. This type of rash is due to the abnormal buildup of the skin protein keratin in the skin follicles. KP seems to be related to allergic diseases, such as atopic dermatitis, allergic rhinitis, and asthma, but it can also occur in people without allergies. It usually does not require treatment and tends to resolve as a child ages. Some people are concerned about the cosmetic appearance of KP; treatment with a variety of over-the-counter moisturizing creams may help, or a prescription cream containing lactic acid (LacHydrin) or tretinoin (Retin-A) may be needed.

Keratosis pilaris (KP)

A skin condition marked by rough, dry bumps on the upper arms, legs, and face, which is often related to allergic diseases.

98. What is contact dermatitis?

Contact dermatitis is a broad term referring to an inflammatory condition of the skin caused by direct contact with an external substance. Irritant contact dermatitis is the most common type of contact dermatitis and involves

Contact dermatitis

A broad term referring to an inflammatory condition of the skin caused by direct contact with an environmental substance.

inflammation resulting from contact with acids, alkaline materials (such as soaps and detergents), solvents, or other chemicals. People who wash their hands repeatedly or wear occlusive gloves for long periods of time may develop intense irritation of the hands. In cases of irritant contact dermatitis, the skin appears dry, red, and chapped.

Allergic contact dermatitis is less common and is caused by exposure to a substance that the person has previously become allergic to, such as poison oak or poison ivy (**Table 10**). As in other types of allergic diseases, repeated exposure to the substance over time is required before allergic contact dermatitis can develop. Following reexposure to the substance, allergic contact reactions usually begin after 12 to 24 hours and reach a peak between 48 and 72 hours after exposure. The skin inflammation in allergic contact dermatitis varies from mild redness and itching to weeping blisters, depending

Table 10   Common Causes of Contact Dermatitis

Allergic Substance	Where It is Found
Urushiol	Poison ivy and poison oak
Nickel	Jewelry, metal snaps
Gold	Jewelry, tooth fillings
Balsam of Peru	Perfumes, skin lotions
Thimerosal	Local antiseptics and in vaccines
Neomycin	First aid creams, cosmetics, deodorants, soaps
Fragrances	Perfumes, cosmetic products, insecticides, antiseptics, soaps, dental products
Formaldehyde	Paper products, paints, medications, household cleaners, cosmetic products, fabrics
Cobalt	Medical products, hair dyes, antiperspirants, metal-plated objects such as snaps, buttons, or tools
Quaternium-15	Self-tanning lotions, shampoos, nail polish, sunscreens, polishes, paints, waxes

on the nature of the substance, the body part affected, and the individual's level of sensitivity.

In addition to plants, the most common causes of allergic contact dermatitis are metals (e.g., nickel), medications (e.g., antibiotics), rubber, and cosmetics. Some products cause a reaction only when they contact the skin and are exposed to sunlight (i.e., photocontact dermatitis). These include shaving lotions, sunscreens, sulfa ointments, some perfumes, and coal tar products. The diagnosis of both irritant and allergic contact dermatitis is primarily based on the history of exposure to an irritant or an allergen and the appearance of the skin. For confirmation purposes, particularly when multiple different substances are suspected, diagnostic patch testing is very useful. The test is performed by applying a series of materials in small patches to the back. The patches are available in a commercial kit or are brought to the doctor's office by the patient. They are removed and the skin is assessed after 48 hours and again at 72 hours, preferably by a clinician with experience in these procedures and interpretation of the results.

99. How should contact dermatitis be treated?

Treatment of irritant contact dermatitis usually involves the cessation of the aggravating activity, initiation of intensive therapy with moisturizers, and if necessary, a short course of topical steroids. Long-term prevention of the rash may be difficult, especially in individuals who repeatedly wash their hands during work, such as nurses and physicians. In these people, use of a moisturizer multiple times throughout the day is extremely important. In people who are in constant contact with irritating chemicals, use of protective gloves is usually needed.

Initial treatment of acute allergic contact dermatitis, such as poison ivy, includes thorough washing with lots of water to remove any trace of the substance that may remain on the skin. If the rash is mild, topical steroids may reduce inflammation and lessen the itching. More severe cases, with pain and blistering over large portions of the body, usually require oral or injected corticosteroids to reduce inflammation. Prednisone is usually given in doses up to 60–80 mg per day, and tapered gradually over 10 to 14 days to prevent recurrence of the rash. Wet dressings, soothing anti-itch or drying lotions (e.g., calamine), and oatmeal baths (e.g., Aveeno-bath) may also provide comfort, particularly when large areas of the skin are involved. With appropriate treatment, acute allergic contact dermatitis usually clears up without complications within 1 to 2 weeks, but it may return if the substance or material that caused it cannot be identified or avoided. It is critical that contact allergens be avoided, and occasionally a change of occupation or alteration of work habits (e.g., use of protective gloves) may be necessary if the rash is caused by occupational exposure.

Treatment of chronic allergic contact dermatitis may be more difficult, as the skin is often hardened and thickened and active inflammation has become less intense. In these patients, complete avoidance of the allergen and aggressive moisturization therapy may be the two most important aspects of the therapeutic program.

Ellen's comment:

I am a nurse in a doctor's office and bring back about 20 to 25 patients per day to be seen by the doctor. Between each patient, I wash my hands with an antibacterial soap and dry them with a paper towel. After working there for about 5 years, I started to notice that my hands were extremely dry and chapped, and occasionally I had cracking between my fingers. I did use latex gloves a couple of times per day to help with procedures, but I never noticed any redness or itching while wearing the gloves or after taking them off. A dermatologist diagnosed me as having irritant contact dermatitis and recommended that I wash only when necessary, use Cetaphil soap while washing, use Nivea cream on my hands while at work, and use Aquaphor ointment in the morning and in the evening. I have been doing this for the past 2 weeks and have seen a marked improvement in my skin.

100. Is it possible to have a skin allergy to sunlight?

A small number of people develop rashes after exposure to sunlight. There are a number of syndromes in which exposure to ultraviolet light, either outdoors or in a tanning salon, results in a rash. Some patients only experience rashes from sun exposure when they are taking an oral medication, such as an antibiotic (**Table 11**).

Table 11   Medications That Cause Drug-Induced Photosensitivity Reactions

Antibiotic
    Tetracycline
    Doxycycline
    Ciprofloxacin
    Sulfonamides

Nonsteroidal anti-inflammatory drugs
    Ibuprofen
    Naproxen

Diuretics
    Furosemide
    Hydrochlorthiazide

HMG Co-A reductase inhibitors
    Statin drugs

Anti-fungals
    Itraconazole
    Voriconazole

The rash often appears as a deep, red sunburn which persists for several days after the sun exposure and may itch or burn. Some patients experience a delayed reaction to sunlight that takes the form of eczema, a condition called polymorphic light eruption. In these patients, some combination of redness, bumps, blistering, and itching typically occurs many hours after sun exposure and may persist for up to a week. Other patients will develop hives within 30 minutes of being in direct sun, which is referred to as solar hives or urticaria. These skin lesions appear like other forms of hives, with itchy welts that resolve within 30 to 60 minutes.

If you have some form of sun sensitivity, you can reduce your risk of a reaction by limiting your time in the sun. One important step is to wear sunglasses, long-sleeved shirts, and wide-brimmed hats while you are outside. If you have solar urticaria, your doctor may recommend the use of oral antihistamines to prevent or reduce a reaction as well as the use of sunscreen. However, sunscreens do not block ultraviolet rays completely, so you may still experience a skin reaction.

American Academy of Allergy, Asthma, and Immunology
www.aaaai.org

Food Allergy and Anaphylaxis Network
www.foodallergy.org

American Academy of Dermatology
www.aad.org

SkinCarePhysicians.com
www.skincarephysicians.com

National Institute of Allergy and Infectious Diseases at the National Institutes of Health
www3.niaid.nih.gov

Acupuncture: The practice of inserting fine needles through the skin at specific points to treat disease or relieve pain.

Acute sinusitis: Inflammation of the mucosal lining of the paranasal sinuses lasting more than 10 days and usually associated with bacterial infection. Antibiotics are generally required for resolution of symptoms.

Allergic conjunctivitis: Inflammation of the conjunctivae of the eye due to an allergic reaction. The conjunctivae is the membrane that covers the front of the eye and extends onto the eyelids.

Allergic rhinitis: Mucosal inflammation of the nose due to an allergic reaction.

Allergy: A type of hypersensitivity reaction to environmental substances caused by IgE antibodies.

Anaphylaxis: A life-threatening allergic reaction most often involving the skin (hives), lungs (wheezing), and circulation (low blood pressure).

Angioedema: Swelling of the deep layers of the skin caused by leakage of fluid from blood vessels into the surrounding tissue.

Antibody: A protein formed by the immune system that helps protect the body from infection and is also responsible for certain types of hypersensitivity reactions.

Antihistamine: An agent that binds to the histamine receptor and blocks the effects of histamine on the body.

Aspirin: A type of nonsteroidal anti-inflammatory drug (NSAID). In addition to pain relief, it is used to prevent heart attacks and strokes.

Asthma: Disease of the lungs in which the bronchial mucous membrane is chronically irritated and inflamed. The hallmarks of this disease include episodic, reversible spasm of the airways in response to both specific (e.g., allergens) and nonspecific (e.g., cold air) triggers.

Atopic dermatitis: A chronic eczematous skin disease characterized by redness, itching, and scaling.

Autism: A neural developmental disorder characterized by impaired social and communication skills.

Autologous serum skin test: Allergy skin test in which a patient's own blood serum is injected into their skin. A positive reaction is most often seen in patients with chronic urticaria and indicates the presence of autoimmune antibodies to certain components in the skin.

Celiac disease: A digestive condition that results from eating gluten, characterized by diarrhea, pain, and intestinal malabsorption.

Chronic idiopathic urticaria: Hives that occur for 6 weeks or longer with no known cause.

Chronic sinusitis: Inflammation of the mucosal lining of the paranasal sinuses that persists for more than 3 months.

Concha bullosa: An air pocket that occurs in the nasal turbinate bones, causing enlargement of the turbinate and often resulting in obstruction to airflow.

Contact dermatitis: A broad term referring to an inflammatory condition of the skin caused by direct contact with an environmental substance.

Cross-contamination: Transfer of a harmful food element from one food product to another, often occurring inadvertently during food production or preparation.

Decongestant: An agent that decreases nasal congestion by constricting blood vessels in the nose.

Drug intolerance: Adverse side effects of a drug that are not mediated by the immune system.

Electrostatic air filter: A filter that places a negative ionic charge upon airborne particles, which then aggregate onto a metal plate in the filter.

Endoscopy: Examination of the body's interior through an instrument inserted into a natural opening or an incision.

Eosinophilic esophagitis: Allergic inflammation that occurs in the esophagus, occasionally as a result of food allergy.

Epinephrine: A naturally occurring hormone that is administered as an injectable drug that is used to stop anaphylactic allergic reactions.

Food hypersensitivity: An adverse immunologic response to a food protein.

Gastroesophageal reflux disease (GERD): A condition in which gastric acid rises from the stomach into the esophagus, causing irritation and inflammation.

High-efficiency particulate air (HEPA) filter: A filter specially designed to remove greater than 90% of small (<1 micron) airborne particles.

Histamine: A compound released during allergic reactions that causes capillary dilation, smooth muscle contraction, and sensory nerve stimulation.

Hives: A skin rash marked by raised, swollen, and itchy patches of skin. Also called urticaria.

Hypoallergenic: A product that manufacturers claim does not contain ingredients known to cause allergic reactions.

Immunoglobulin E (IgE): The antibody that is responsible for allergic responses.

Immunologic sensitivity: Sensitivity to a substance which is caused by components of the immune system, including antibodies and lymphocytes

Immunotherapy: A form of treatment for allergic diseases in which the patient receives increasing amounts of the substance that they are allergic to, resulting in tolerance.

Intradermal skin test: An allergy test in which an allergen extract is injected into the skin.

Keratosis pilaris (KP): A skin condition marked by rough, dry bumps on the upper arms, legs, and face, which is often related to allergic diseases.

Lactose intolerance: Inability to digest lactose, which is a principal sugar of milk, which causes symptoms of diarrhea, abdominal pain, and bloating.

Leukotriene: A family of lipid molecules, which are released during allergic reactions and whose most prominent effects are tissue swelling and bronchoconstriction.

Mast cell: A type of tissue cell rich in histamine, which is the major cause of immediate allergic reactions.

Nasal polyp: A growth that usually originates in the mucous membrane of the sinus cavity and extends into the nose.

Nasal septum: The small cartilaginous structure that divides the nose into halves.

Nonallergic rhinitis: Nasal inflammatory disease that is not caused by IgE-mediated hypersensitivity to allergens.

Occupational rhinitis: Rhinitis that is associated with an individual's work environment.

Oral allergy syndrome: A food allergy to certain raw fruits and vegetables that causes itching and occasionally swelling of the oral cavity.

Otitis media with effusion: Inflammation of the middle ear with resultant fluid collection in the middle ear space.

Paranasal sinuses: The air-filled spaces within the bones of the skull and face.

Prick/puncture skin test: Allergy test in which the most superficial layer of skin is pricked or punctured with an allergen extract.

Prostaglandin: A family of lipid molecules derived from arachidonic acid whose effects include tissue inflammation.

Radiocontrast medium (RCM): Dye injected into a person to improve visibility of internal structures during an x-ray procedure (e.g., intravenous pyelogram for detection of kidney stones).

Radioimmunosorbent test (RAST): A type of blood allergy test in which IgE antibodies to specific allergens are measured.

Rhinitis medicamentosa: Rebound nasal congestion brought on by extended use of topical nasal decongestants.

Turbinate: A long, narrow, and curled bone that comes off of the lateral wall of the nasal passage and is important in the humidification, filtration, and warming of inspired air.

Urticaria: See *hives*.

Vasodilation: The widening of blood vessels.

Page numbers followed by "*f*" and "*t*" represent figures and tables, respectively.

Index